CASE STUDIES IN PUBLIC HEALTH ETHICS

D1128987

STEVEN S. COUGHLIN, PH.D.

COLIN L. SOSKOLNE, PH.D.

KENNETH W. GOODMAN, PH.D.

Case Studies in Public Health Ethics

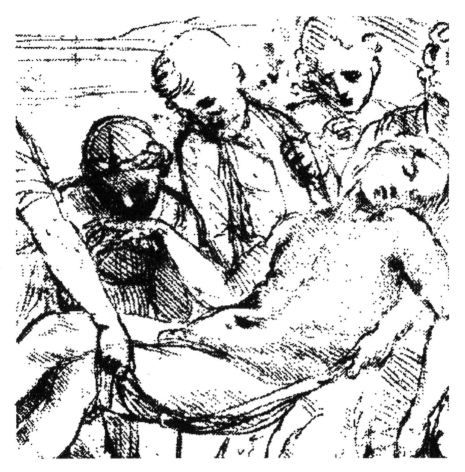

STEVEN S. COUGHLIN, PH.D.

COLIN L. SOSKOLNE, PH.D.

KENNETH W. GOODMAN, PH.D.

AMERICAN PUBLIC HEALTH ASSOCIATION
WASHINGTON, DC

Copyright © 1997 by the American Public Health Association

AMERICAN PUBLIC HEALTH ASSOCIATION
800 I Street, NW
Washington, DC 20001-3710

Mohammad N. Akhter, MD, MPH
Executive Director

Library of Congress card catalog number 97-76770.

ISBN: 0-87553-232-2

2M 9/97
5C 8/03
5C 12/04
1M 7/05

Printed and bound in the United States of America
Typesetting: Marilyn Butler
Set in: Palatino
Cover Design by Sam Dixon, Dixon Design Studio.
Printing: United Book Press, Inc., Baltimore, Md.

TABLE OF CONTENTS

PREFACE

S everal individuals who have taught courses on public health ethics over the past few years have observed that there is a pressing need for case study materials that illustrate ethical concerns and problems in public health research and practice. Such materials are an instrumental part of case-based methods of instruction in public health ethics, both in graduate degree programs and in continuing professional education programs such as those offered by the American College of Epidemiology and the International Society for Environmental Epidemiology. This book of edited case studies is an attempt to fill that gap so that public health ethics can be more readily taught and learned.

Our objective is to provide students and instructors with a compilation of case studies in public health ethics suitable for classroom discussions and professional workshops. Although challenges arising in epidemiology figure prominently, the focus of the book is much broader and encompasses many other areas of public health research and practice. This seems appropriate since epidemiology is the science that provides the rational basis for public health policy and practice.

This book is organized into 16 chapters. Chapter 1 provides an overview of methods of moral reasoning suitable for analyzing ethical problems in public health. The chapters that follow deal with issues of privacy and confidentiality protection, informed consent in public health research, the ethics of randomized trials, the institutional review board system, scientific misconduct, conflicting interests, and intellectual property and data sharing.

Emerging issues in public health ethics are covered. They include the publication and interpretation of research findings and the communication responsibilities of public health professionals. Ethical issues in public health practice are also addressed. Other chapters deal with ethical issues in studies of vulnerable populations, cross-cultural research, genetic discrimination, HIV/AIDS prevention and treatment, and health care reform and the allocation of scarce resources. While the cases are drawn from the fields of public health and epidemiology, many issues will be recognized by those familiar with the burgeoning literature on research integrity and the responsible conduct of science. The annotated case studies presented in each chapter are accompanied by questions for further reflection along with extensive references. An instructor's guide is provided at the end.

Finally, a note about usage. We have used the phrase "study participants" rather than the less respectful term "subjects," although we recognize that the latter is widely used in the bioethics literature with good intentions.

We welcome comments on any aspect of this book that might benefit future editions.

Steven S. Coughlin, PhD
Tulane University[*]

Colin L. Soskolne, PhD
University of Alberta

Kenneth W. Goodman, PhD
University of Miami

[*]*Present Affiliation: Centers for Disease Control and Prevention*

ACKNOWLEDGMENTS

W e are indebted to the members of the American Public Health Association Publications Board for their thoughtful comments on a preliminary outline of this book. We also benefited from many stimulating discussions with professional colleagues, including faculty and students at Tulane University, the University of Michigan at Ann Arbor, the University of Alberta, and the University of Miami. Lee Sieswerda and Lee-Anne Hatten worked closely with Colin L. Soskolne in developing case studies from an international ethics survey of environmental epidemiologists. Their insights and creativity are much appreciated. Lee-Anne Hatten was supported by an Alberta Heritage Foundation for Medical Research 1996 Summer Studentship. Catherine Metayer also served as a capable and energetic research assistant. Much assistance was provided by the medical center libraries at our respective institutions. We would especially like to thank Sabine Beisler and Shiriki Kumanyika for assisting us with this project.

Many of the case studies contributed to this book by Colin L. Soskolne were made possible by participants in the International Society for Environmental Epidemiology, the Global Environmental Epidemiology NETWORK of the World Health Organization, and the Italian Epidemiology Association 1994 International Ethics Survey. We are indebted to those respondents who were kind enough to provide at least one case study and to allow them to be included in a book of case studies for teaching purposes. The preliminary results of the International Ethics Survey were published in the May 17, 1996, issue of *The Science of the Total Environment*. Three case studies were developed by Gina Etheredge, Judith La Rosa, and Ronald Prineas for teaching purposes and are included here in revised form with the kind permission of the authors.

Chapter 1

Case Analysis and Moral Reasoning

P ublic health research and practice raise a variety of important ethical issues. These issues have inspired a significant increase in efforts to examine and clarify the rights and responsibilities of practitioners, investigators, study participants, communities, and governments.

Many of these efforts relate to the identification of ethical issues and core values in epidemiology and other areas of public health. Additionally, there is increasing interest in the development of ethics guidelines or professional codes of conduct for epidemiologists as public health professionals. Guidelines and codes are useful for educational purposes, for some dispute resolution, and to guide behavior in relatively clear-cut cases; however, they do not provide specific answers to many of the complex ethical questions encountered in public health research and practice. Public health professionals therefore need to be skilled at ethical decision making so they can make and justify decisions in their own professional pursuits. It is clear that most public health professionals are not experts in moral philosophy; conversely, moral philosophers are rarely experts in public health disciplines.

Public health professionals need to be familiar with at least some methods of moral reasoning, and there has been vigorous debate in the recent bioethics literature over alternative approaches to moral reasoning. Competing approaches that have been defended include the principle-based approach of Beauchamp and Childress (1994), case-based or analogical methods such as casuistry (Jonsen and Toulmin, 1988), and moral rule-based systems (Gert, 1988). One could add to this list rights-based theories; duty-based theories; contractarianism; virtue ethics;

1

and more recent developments in bioethics such as the ethics of care, narrative ethics, and communitarianism or community-based theories, although a detailed explication of these various approaches to moral reasoning is beyond the scope of this text. Obviously, it is impractical for the vast majority of public health professionals to master such diverse theoretical frameworks in order to identify and solve ethical problems in public health research and practice.

In deciding which conceptual or analytical frameworks to emphasize in this introductory chapter, we were guided by theoretical considerations and by the need for practicality and applicability to actual moral problems in public health. In the discussion that follows, a brief overview of ethical theories is provided, along with an introduction to three of the leading methods of ethical decision making. They are the four-principles approach, casuistry, and rule-based morality.

This account should not be mistaken for a complete or comprehensive introduction to the tools needed for ethical decision making. It is offered as a brief introduction to concepts that are best taught with somewhat greater philosophical depth and rigor. The question of how much depth and rigor is itself a topic debated among those who teach applied ethics to professionals.

Overview of Ethical Theories

Moral reasoning involves deliberating about ethical questions and problems and coming to a decision with the help of judgment or rational analysis. In such deliberations we sometimes seek to justify particular decisions and actions by applying moral rules and principles, which are in turn justified by ethical theory. A decision or action and the ethical rules and principles used to make it, may be defended by an ethical theory, or by an integrated body of rules and principles.

Deontological and utilitarian theories, two commonly cited theories, have relevance to public health ethics. Deontological or Kantian theories hold that individuals should not be treated simply as means to an end and that some actions are right or wrong regardless of their consequences. Deontology provides strong support for protecting participants in research that uses human subjects, even if such protections slow research or the acquisition of knowledge.

Utilitarian theories, on the other hand, strive to maximize beneficial consequences. To utilitarians, the principle of utility (which requires the maximization of aggregate or collective benefits) is the ultimate ethical principle from which all other principles are derived. Utilitarian theories provide strong justification for public health programs such as compulsory vaccination programs, the fluoridation of public water supplies, and the collection of vital statistics.

To determine their adequacy, moral theories can be tested for completeness, comprehensiveness, and congruence with ordinary moral judgments and experience (Beauchamp and Childress, 1994). It is extraordinarily difficult to satisfy all these requirements, which may reflect the complexity of morality (Lustig, 1992). As Beauchamp and Childress put it, "We develop theories to illuminate experience and to determine what we ought to do, but we also use experience to test, corroborate, and revise theories. If a theory yields conclusions at odds with our ordinary judgments—for example, if it allows human subjects to be used merely as means to the ends of scientific research—we have reason to be suspicious of the theory and to modify it or seek an alternative theory" (Beauchamp and Childress, 1994).

Principle-Based Methods of Moral Reasoning

Ethical rules and guidelines for public health can be formulated by referring to the principles of beneficence, nonmaleficence, autonomy, and justice, although the rules and guidelines cannot be deduced directly from the principles. These principles, which form the core of the approach developed by Beauchamp and Childress (1994), seek to reduce morality to its basic elements and to provide a useful framework for ethical analysis in the health professions. They do not provide a full philosophical justification for decision making, however. Such abstract principles and other general norms provide only nonspecific advice and often are open to competing interpretations. In situations where there is conflict or tension between principles such as beneficence and justice or nonmaleficence and autonomy, it may be necessary to choose between principles or to assign greater weight to a particular principle. Practical problems in public health ethics require that these principles be made more suitably applicable through a process of specification and reform.

Ethical principles. The principles of beneficence, nonmaleficence, autonomy, and justice provide a framework for applying normative ethics to moral problems in public health. The ethical principle of beneficence requires that potential benefits to individuals and to society be maximized and that potential harms be minimized. Beneficence involves both the protection of the welfare of individuals and the promotion of the common welfare (Beauchamp and Childress, 1994).

The principle of nonmaleficence—which has been associated with the Hippocratic injunction to do no harm—requires that harmful acts not be committed. However, the principle of nonmaleficence does not preclude balancing potential harms against potential benefits.

The principle of justice requires the equitable distribution of potential benefits and burdens. Several theories of distributive justice have been put forth. An egalitarian theory of justice holds that each person in society should receive an equal share of potential benefits. Utilitarian theories of justice, on the other hand, emphasize a mixture of criteria so that public utility is maximized; this approach resembles the way public health policy has often been formulated. A utilitarian theory determines just distribution of health resources by their utility to all affected. In contrast, libertarian theories of justice emphasize rights to social and economic liberty; these theories hold that distributions of health care services and goods are best left to the marketplace. In a true free market, resources are allocated through individual choice and enterprise rather than through central or government planning. (Issues of distributive justice are further discussed in Chapter 16.)

Finally, the principle of autonomy focuses on the right of self-determination. Respect for persons is a principle rooted in the Western tradition, which grants importance to individual freedom in political life and personal development. Several ideas loosely associated with autonomy include privacy, choosing freely, and accepting responsibility for one's choices.

Further specification and interpretation of general norms and principles is essential to the resolution of ethical problems. In difficult cases, the first step is to specify general norms and to reduce or resolve conflicts through further specification and reform (Beauchamp, 1996). Specification makes principles less general and therefore potentially more applicable. Progressive specification is then needed on an ongoing basis as new problems arise.

To illustrate how the four-principles approach can be used to analyze a specific problem in public health, consider the following ethical challenge.

Case 1a. An epidemiologist at a university in the United States was asked to undertake an industry-sponsored study of miscarriages among female fabrication workers at several semiconductor manufacturing plants. A research protocol drafted by the researcher was approved by the Institutional Review Board (also known as an Ethics Review Committee) at his university. The contract for the study, which did not address issues of publication, was signed by both the epidemiologist and the company's administrative officer. The contract stipulated that all materials and information gleaned by the research team were to remain company property.

The epidemiologist enlisted the help of a team of epidemiology graduate students. The researchers found that exposure to a range of chemicals used in part of the manufacturing process was associated with increased rates of miscarriages and infertility. The results and recommendations were submitted to the company head office, but were not published in the scientific literature.

The trade union representing the workers inquired about the findings after some of its members participated in the study by completing lifestyle questionnaires and medical histories. The union unsuccessfully petitioned the company for the research results. Subsequently, the union contacted the university-based epidemiologist and asked him for the results. The researcher was told by the company head office that he was not permitted to release his results under the terms of the contractual agreement.

Under threat of legal action, he felt compelled to withhold the findings from the trade union and from the workers employed by the company.

Example of principle-based analysis. The epidemiologist who undertook the study was faced with a difficult professional and ethical challenge. The ethical principle of beneficence requires that the epidemiologist minimize potential risks to the fabrication workers and their families, and that the potential benefits of the study, both to the workers and to society in general, be maximized. The need to reduce or prevent harm to future workers, as required by the principles of beneficence and nonmaleficence, also must be taken into account. Thus, the epidemiologist has a professional obligation to disclose the research findings in a timely fashion so that the widest possible audience stands to benefit from the research.

The principle of autonomy suggests that the fabrication workers have a right to be fully informed about the risks associated with employment in the semiconductor industry. The principle of justice also suggests that women suffering miscarriages or infertility as a result of exposure to industrial chemicals are entitled to compensation for their injuries.

Nevertheless, the epidemiologist should respect the law and honor his contractual agreements by protecting the confidentiality of privileged information. Failure to honor the agreement might place him in legal difficulty and reduce financial support for future research from industry sources. By disclosing the results of the study, the epidemiologist also could expose the industrial sponsor of the research to possible financial losses and legal liability. Thus, legal and financial risks to the epidemiologist and to the industrial sponsor must be balanced against potential benefits to the female fabrication workers and the need to protect them from harm.

To reduce conflicts between ethical principles and related normative rules (such as "protect the confidentiality of privileged information"), the principles must be further specified and interpreted. Under some circumstances, for example, the need to inform workers about serious risks to their health may carry greater weight than the general need to honor contractual agreements. Other possible resolutions to this ethical dilemma include persuading company officials to agree to allow the epidemiologist to release his results to the trade union or to publish them in the scientific literature. History suggests that when companies suppress important research findings about industrial health risks, they often expose themselves to future legal liability and may eventually be obligated to pay compensatory damages. The epidemiologist also could seek legal assistance to scrutinize the perceived threat of legal action. On closer inspection, he might not be legally obliged to withhold the study findings from the trade union and its workers.

The epidemiologist's apparent inability to disclose his research findings to the workers or to publish them in the scientific literature is a result of conflicting interests. Safeguards are needed to ensure that such conflicting interests do not occur when university-based scientists conduct research on behalf of industry. Institutional policies and ethics guidelines should deter researchers from entering into contractual agreements that prevent them from disclosing their research findings to study participants or publishing them in the scientific literature.

On balance, we believe the four principles provide stronger support for informing workers about the exposure risk than for withholding this information. While legal concerns need to be taken into account, moral obligation is generally regarded to supersede fears of liability, financial risk, and so forth. What this means is that doing the right thing sometimes produces consequences we would otherwise hope to avoid. This conflict and concern could have been prevented had the original contract ensured reasonable rights for the scientist to publish his findings.

Despite the appeal of principle-based methods, there has been important debate in the bioethics literature over methods of moral reasoning. Several alternatives to principle-based methods have been proposed, including methods based upon analogical reasoning such as casuistry.

Casuistry and Analogical Reasoning

Casuistry (the Latin root means "case") originated with the ancient Stoics and achieved prominence in the 15th and 16th centuries in the work of Roman Catholic and Anglican moral theologians (Jonsen and Toulmin, 1988; Jonsen, 1995). It came to be a term of derision used to designate quibbling or faulty reasoning. The method—and the term—have been rehabilitated and invigorated by the philosophers Albert Jonsen, Stephen Toulmin, and others.

Casuistry is founded on analogical reasoning, appeal to paradigmatic cases, and practical judgment. Jonsen argues that while many general ethical questions have been answered on the basis of general principles and theories, the specific decisions that emerge in particular cases remain unaddressed by the principles. He contends that such decisions are made by focusing on the circumstances of the case at hand and the moral context in which the case rests.

In casuistry, decision making takes place at the level of the particulars of the case itself. Given a case and a particular decision to be made, a casuist need not refer directly to a particular theory. Rather, one identifies maxims—wise, pithy, rulelike sayings, such as "tell the truth," that have bearing on the case. A case usually involves several maxims.

Casuistry requires a clear exposition of the circumstances of a case, i.e., the facts that surround it. There can be more or fewer of these facts, depending on the completeness of the description. The casuist then must decide which maxim is the most appropriate to "rule" or govern the case. Differing circumstances or facts might require emphasizing a different maxim. The casuist then makes a claim regarding the case—a judgment. The claim is backed by a form of logical reasoning described in terms of grounds (the relevant circumstances), maxims, and the backings (more general notions, such as respect for persons, that support the maxims).

The description of the case, which includes circumstances, maxims, and logical thought, constitutes its basic structure or *morphology*. Placing a particular case alongside other similar cases constitutes *taxonomy*, and moving from case to case within these structures is what Jonsen refers to as *kinetics*.

Casuists begin with relatively clear, paradigmatic cases in which some ethical norm indicates the right course of action. Judgment is necessary to determine which norm applies in a complicated or ambiguous case. Casuistry proceeds much like the application of law which is based upon precedent-setting cases.

Consider the following case presentation as an illustration of the casuistic method.

Case 1b. A provocative hypothesis that sunscreens may paradoxically increase the risk of malignant melanoma has been widely reported in the news media. The hypothesis was proposed by three California epidemiologists and is based largely on correlational data and other indirect evidence (Garland et al., 1992). Rigorous epidemiologic studies designed to test this hypothesis have not been published in peer-reviewed journals. The hypothesis is based upon the following observations:

• Rising rates of malignant melanoma have been roughly paralleled by increases in the marketing and use of sunscreens.

• There is no conclusive scientific evidence that sunscreens help prevent melanoma. Public health recommendations about the use of sunscreens for preventing skin cancer are largely untested.

• Sunscreens block ultraviolet B (UVB) radiation, which causes sunburn, but (at least until recently) are transparent to UVA radiation, which has been shown to be carcinogenic in animals.

• By blocking UVB radiation, sunscreens inhibit the production of vitamin D. Vitamin D may prevent certain cancers in humans including melanoma, breast cancer, and colon cancer.

The epidemiologists who proposed this hypothesis are concerned that individuals who use sunscreens may have acquired a false sense of security. They point out that, because sunscreen users tend not to burn when exposed to sunlight, they may have excessive exposure to potentially carcinogenic wavelengths of sunlight. The epidemiologists caution that sunscreen users may actually be increasing their risk of malignant melanoma. Instead of sunscreen, they recommend traditional measures to reduce sunlight exposure, such as limiting time spent in the sun or the use of protective clothing. The hypothesis has generated scientific and medical controversy.

Example of case-based analysis. In analyzing this case, the casuist first considers its circumstances, i.e., the facts surrounding it (indeed, this is crucial for any ethics analysis). These include the fact that the hypothesis was based largely upon correlational data, the lack of conclusive scientific evidence that sunscreens help prevent melanoma, the fact that public health recommendations about the use of sunscreens for preventing skin cancer are largely untested, and the like.

The casuist also must decide which maxims are the most appropriate to rule the case. Maxims in this case could be that "epidemiologists and other public health professionals should not communicate untested hypotheses to the general public through the news media" or "the public has a right to information about preliminary health research results." Other maxims could include "research findings should be released to the public only after they have undergone rigorous peer review;" "public health professionals must ensure that research findings are presented to the public in an objective and thoughtful fashion;" "the communication of scientific information to lay persons should not be entirely left up to journalists;" "the deliberate withholding or nondisclosure of health information is overly paternalistic and is never justified in public health."

The basic structure of this enriched case is then considered in light of previous cases and narratives that relate to the communication responsibilities of public health professionals and their interactions with the media. The casuist emphasizes particularly clear or paradigmatic cases in which the right course of action was clearly discernible.

The casuist then makes a claim regarding the case, namely that the public should (or should not) be alerted to possible risks from sunscreen usage, given the current scientific uncertainty. As Weed (1996) has explained, "This claim is, in essence, the judgment of the individual using the casuist's method, and it is backed by maxims which are in turn supported by more general notions... One such general notion could be, for example, the weighing of risks and benefits found within the principle of beneficence."

This analysis seems to point to the following conclusion: Scientists must include scrutiny of the public consequences of scientific reporting. In rare instances, researchers might consider delaying or forgoing publication. In the case at hand, the epidemiologists should take pains to be available to journalists, so that they can make clear the nature of the correlation and caution strongly against conclusions or surmises that outstrip available evidence.

As Last (1996: 59) observed:

Epidemiologic findings are sometimes open to misinterpretation if presented carelessly or without caveat. In our dealings with the media, we must not sensationalize: we should make conscious efforts to present the facts objectively and with sufficient explanation to ensure that the news reaching the general public does not mislead either by unnecessarily arousing alarm or by falsely reassuring people that their way of life is conducive to longevity.

As the above case study illustrates, casuistry can provide an account of the source of our intuitive understanding of particular cases, that is, traditions and practices. Casuistry also seems to be an interesting account of how moral understanding is acquired (DeGrazia, 1992). On the other hand, casuistry has been criticized for its excessive reliance on intuitive judgments in cases of conflict. A further limitation is that global ethical issues may be missed in focusing solely on specific cases (DeGrazia, 1992). Thus, the advantages and disadvantages of alternative methods of moral reasoning must be considered in any comprehensive course on public health ethics.

Moral Rules and Ideals

An important alternative to principle-based or analogical approaches is the theory of morality developed by the philosopher Bernard Gert (1988). Gert argues that contemporary bioethics attends too much to difficult cases when, in fact, there is broad if not universal agreement on many moral judgments. A comprehensive theory of morality is a public system that must capture the key features of those judgments. To advocate evil is irrational, according to Gert, and rationality is the fundamental normative concept. Correspondingly, it is rational to avoid harms. Consider the following definitions.

Rationality and Irrationality:

An essential feature of the actions I classify as irrational, or rationally prohibited, is that everyone will agree that they are actions that they would never advocate to anyone for whom they were concerned; on the contrary, they would advocate that these persons always avoid performing such actions (Gert, 1988: 19f).

Evils and Goods:

Everyone agrees that death and pain are evils... the desires for pain or death are irrational desires. Since desires for death and pain are irrational desires and since death and pain are evils, it is plausible that there is a close relationship between the objects of irrational desires and evils ... I shall attempt to show the advantages of defining an evil as the object of an irrational desire (p. 48).

Although the absence of evils is the only thing we are certain that all rational persons desire, we know that there are many other things which no rational person would avoid without a reason. We can therefore define *a good as that which no rational person will avoid without a reason* (p. 50).

Moral Rules:

... the moral rules, or at least the most important basic moral rules, share a set of characteristics that distinguishes them from all other rules ... these characteristics enable them to form the core of a public system that applies to all rational persons, such that all impartial persons would advocate adopting that system (p. 62).

There are 10 moral rules: Don't kill, don't cause pain, don't disable, don't deprive of freedom, don't deprive of pleasure, don't deceive, keep your promise, don't cheat, obey the law, do your duty.

Moral Ideals: "The most important moral ideals are directly concerned with lessening of such evils as death, pain, and disability..." (p. 161). "As long as an impartial person can publicly allow it, any action that seeks to lessen the amount of evil in the world is encouraged by the moral ideals" (p. 178).

From the definitions, the following emerges: The moral rules identify morally salient or relevant features of instances in which moral judgments are called for. The right thing to do in such situations will be determined in part by whether a rational person could publicly advocate the action. The following case presentation illustrates Gert's system.

Case 1c. Investigators want to test banked blood or tissue samples which have been routinely collected from a group of patients to study the prevalence of the BRCA1 breast cancer genetic marker. They also want to be able to prospectively follow the individuals from whom the samples have been obtained, so that they can look at associations with specific causes of death. This means that each tissue sample will need to be linked to some unique identifier (e.g., a Social Security number) and to the information gleaned from the tests. The investigators believe it will be difficult, if not impossible, to obtain informed consent from all the patients, and that even if it were easy, many patients might not want the tests performed on their blood or tissue. Because the investigators do not intend to reveal the test results to anyone, except in aggregate form in scientific publications, they argue that they should be allowed to conduct the tests without informing the individuals from whom the blood or tissue was obtained.

Example of moral rule-based analysis. To fail to inform the patients of the testing is to deceive them, because the test was not disclosed when the blood or tissue samples were obtained. Silence, like lying, can constitute deception, namely the production of a false belief in another or the allowing of circumstances in which another has a false belief.

But "do not deceive" is one of the moral rules, which means in part that any rational, impartial person would publicly advocate following it. To be sure, there are circumstances in which it is morally permissible to deceive, namely those situations in which an impartial, rational person would publicly advocate the deception. (Imagine remaining silent or lying when asked by a kidnapper for the whereabouts of a person he intends to abduct.) Thus, in some cases, public advocacy of deception might make sense if the deception produces benefits or reduces harms. But deception also erodes trust, and so might, in the longer run, actually increase harm. In other words, it is sometimes permissible to break a rule, but such situations are rare and require additional justification.

Now, the investigators might argue that the benefits to society would be significant if they could acquire knowledge about the prevalence and etiologic role of the BRCA1 marker. Is this sufficient to warrant deception? It seems that it is not. Most any rational person would want to know that tissue samples provided for clinical diagnosis, for instance, were later used for another purpose. One might simply want to learn the results of the later genetic tests. But it would not be irrational *not* to want to learn the results. Neither position can be determined independently of asking the patients—precisely what the investigators are loathe to do. This means that it is hard to imagine that a rational, impartial person would publicly advocate testing on linked tissue samples without consent. In other words, such testing would be unethical. (For a complete account of the application of Gert's theory of morality to cases in genetics, see Gert et al. [1996]).

Summary and Conclusions

Decisions about which method or methods of moral reasoning to employ can be made on the basis of practicality and applicability to actual ethical problems in public health as well as on the basis of theoretical considerations. Most discussion and debate over alternative approaches in bioethics has focused on clinical practice in medicine, nursing, and psychology. It is not yet clear which approaches or methods are best suited for public health ethics. We find that the three approaches sketched here can each be of use in the analysis of ethical issues in public health, at least in principle. A comprehensive philosophical assessment is required to test the various methods against the kinds of problems and challenges that are (more or less) distinctive to public health.

Public health professionals ought nevertheless to have some understanding of the concepts and language of ethics and at least a rudimentary understanding of major moral traditions. The tension between Kantian and utilitarian perspectives is a familiar one in public health. Nevertheless, as Beauchamp (1996) has pointed out, some perspective is needed on the limitations of moral philosophy and ethical theory as sources for our judgments in public health ethics.

The analysis of case studies, such as those included in this book, is a useful means of clarifying ethics concepts in public health research and practice. As Brody (1990) has put it, "Sometimes what is needed to bring out the significance of a problem which heretofore has not been adequately discussed is one good case study. A case study that highlights the significance of the issue and the need for further discussion will then be a case study of significance and value." Moreover, good case presentations illuminate the way in which a variety of different ethical questions interact with each other within the particular facts of a case. In this way, case studies call attention to real ethical questions in public health that might otherwise be neglected.

Although we favor "real-life" ethical case studies, like those included in this book, over hypothetical or fictional ones, we have no doubt introduced our own subtle biases and perspectives in constructing and interpreting these narratives. As Chambers (1996: 25) explains:

> For the ethicist to present the data received from real life situations, he or she must present those events in a narrative; a story must be constructed. Every telling of a story—real or imagined—encompasses a series of choices about what will be revealed, what will be privileged, and what will be concealed; there are no artless narrations.

All narratives (including ethics case studies) are, Chambers suggests, shaped by the storyteller for a specific purpose, even though they are based upon actual events.

In the chapters that follow, difficult problems in public health ethics are described and accompanied by study questions suggesting possible areas for analysis, reflection, and debate. That reasonable people may disagree about the solutions to individual cases is one of the things that makes applied ethics so exciting and instructive for students. We will have achieved our goal if we foster some of that excitement and creative thinking in students and practitioners of the public health professions.

There is a sense in which both public health and applied ethics aim at prevention. Despite the ancient debate over whether virtue can be taught, it is neither naive nor overly optimistic to suppose that ethics education (including the use of case studies) could have a salutary effect on behavior. At least, students and practitioners can become better aware of what constitutes a clear case of wrongdoing. It is our hope that ethics education will stimulate critical thinking which, in turn, will improve decision making. To the extent that ethics education can prevent harm and reduce wrongs, it serves as a valuable goal and one to which this volume aspires.

References

Beauchamp, T. L. (1994). The "four-principles" approach. In R. Gillon (Ed.), *Principles of health care ethics* (pp. 3-12). New York: John Wiley & Sons.

Beauchamp, T. L. (1995). Principlism and its alleged competitors. *Kennedy Inst Ethics J*, 5, 181-188.

Beauchamp, T. L. (1996). Moral foundations. In S. S. Coughlin & T. L. Beauchamp (Eds.), *Ethics and epidemiology* (pp. 24-52). New York: Oxford University Press.

Beauchamp, T. L. & Childress, J. F. (1994). *Principles of biomedical ethics* (4th ed). New York: Oxford University Press.

Brody, B. A. (1990). Quality of scholarship in bioethics. *J Med Phil*, 15, 161-178.

Chambers, T. (1996). From the ethicist's point of view. The literary nature of ethical inquiry. *Hastings Center Rep*, 26, 25-32.

DeGrazia, D. (1992). Moving forward in bioethical theory: Theories, cases, and specified principlism. *J Med Philos*, 17, 511-539.

Garland, C. F., Garland, F. C. & Gorham, E. D. (1992) Could sunscreens increase melanoma risk? [Letter]. *Am J Public Health*, 82, 614-615.

Gert, B. (1988). *Morality: A new justification of the moral rules.* New York: Oxford University Press.

Gert, B., Berger, E. M., Cahill, G. F., et al. (1996). *Morality and the new genetics: A guide for students and health care providers.* Boston: Jones and Bartlett.

Jonsen, A. R. (1995). Casuistry: an alternative or complement to principles? *Kennedy Inst Ethics J,* 5, 237-251.

Jonsen, A. R. & Toulmin, S. E. (1988). *The abuse of casuistry.* Berkeley, CA: University of California Press.

Last, J. (1996). Professional standards of conduct for epidemiologists. In S.S. Coughlin & T. L. Beauchamp (Eds.), *Ethics and epidemiology* (pp. 53-75). New York: Oxford University Press.

Lustig, B. A. (1992). The method of "principlism": A critique of the critique. *J Med Philos,* 17, 487-510.

Weed, D. L. (1996). Epistemology and ethics in epidemiology. In S. S. Coughlin & T. L. Beauchamp (Eds). *Ethics and epidemiology* (pp. 76-94). New York: Oxford University Press.

Weed, D. L. & Coughlin, S. S. (1995). Ethics in cancer prevention and control. In P. Greenwald, B. F. Kramer, D. L. Weed (Eds.), *Cancer prevention and control* (pp. 497-507). New York: Marcel-Dekker.

Suggestions for Further Reading

Arras, J. D. (1994). Principles and particularity: The role of cases in bioethics. *Indiana Law J,* 69, 983-1014.

Arras, J. D. (1991). Getting down to cases: The revival of casuistry in bioethics. *J Med Philos,* 16, 29-51.

Beauchamp, T. L. (1994). Principles and other emerging paradigms in bioethics. *Indiana Law J,* 69, 955-971.

Beauchamp, T. L. (1993). The principles approach. *Hastings Center Rep,* 23, S9.

Beauchamp, T. L. & Walters, L. (1994) . Ethical theory and bioethics. In *Contemporary issues in bioethics* (4th ed) (pp. 1-38). Belmont, CA: Wadsworth.

Brody, H. (1994). The four principles and narrative ethics. In R. Gillon (Ed.). *Principles of health care ethics.* New York: John Wiley & Sons.

Childress, J. F. (1994). Ethical theories, principles, and casuistry in bioethics: An interpretation and defense of principlism. In P. F. Camenisch (Ed.), *Religious methods and resources in bioethics*. Boston, MA: Kluwer Academic.

Clouser, K. D. (1995). Common morality as an alternative to principlism. *Kennedy Inst Ethics J*, 5, 219-236.

Clouser, K. D. & Gert, B. (1990). A critique of principlism. *J Med Philos*, 15, 219-236.

Clouser, K. D. & Gert, B. (1994). Morality vs. principlism. In R. Gillon (Ed.). *Principles of health care ethics* . New York: John Wiley & Sons, 1994.

DuBose, E. R., Hamel, R. P. & O'Connell, L.J. (Eds.). (1994). *A matter of principles? Ferment in U.S. bioethics*. Valley Forge, PA: Trinity Press International.

Green, R. M., Gert, B. & Clouser, K. D. (1993). The method of public morality versus the method of principlism. *J Med Philos*, 18, 179-197.

Jonsen, A. (1986). Casuistry and clinical ethics. *Theoretical Med*, 7, 67-71.

Jonsen, A. R. (1991). Casuistry as methodology in clinical ethics. *Theoretical Med*, 12, 299-302.

Koppelman, L. M. (1994). Case method and casuistry: The problem of bias. *Theoretical Med*, 15, 21-37.

Singer, P. (Ed.). (1994). *A companion to ethics*. Cambridge, MA: Blackwell Publishers.

Soskolne, C. L. (1991). Ethical decision-making in epidemiology: The case study approach. *J Clin Epidemiol*, 44,(Suppl. I), 125S-130S.

Soskolne, C. L. (1991). Rationalizing professional conduct: Ethics in disease control. *Public Health Review*, 19, 311-321.

Soskolne, C. L. (1989). Epidemiology: Questions of science, ethics, morality, and law. *Am J Epidemiol*, 129, 1-18.

Soskolne, C. L. (1985). Epidemiological research, interest groups and the review process. *J Public Health Policy*, 6, 173-184.

Toulmin, S. (1981). The tyranny of principles. *Hastings Center Rep*, 11, 31-39.

Winkler, E. R. (1996). Reflections on the relevance of the Georgetown paradigm for the ethics of environmental epidemiology. *The Science of the Total Environment*, 184, 113-120.

Chapter 2

Protection of Privacy and Confidentiality

Notions about what constitutes personal or private information vary somewhat over time and from culture to culture. In many societies today, sensitive information includes one's income, certain diseases, sexual habits or orientation, and so forth. With advances in genetic technology, the ability to identify genotypes possibly predisposing to premature illness or death also raises concerns about privacy and confidentiality.

There are many reasons why individuals might wish to have their privacy respected or to have information about themselves held in confidence. Some individuals might fear discrimination simply because they have an attribute, lifestyle, or marker for disease that is stigmatized in society. For example, it was discovered early on in the AIDS epidemic that an AIDS diagnosis could result in loss of employment or residence, or social ostracism. Mental illness also may result in discrimination or social isolation. Genetic discrimination also is of concern as discussed in Chapter 14.

Public health researchers must meet their professional obligations and secure the participation of the individuals they study by rigorously protecting the confidentiality of collected information. Measures that may be taken to protect individual privacy and ensure the confidentiality of health information include keeping records with personal identifiers under lock and key, limiting access to confidential records to selected members of the research team on a need-to-know basis, discarding personal identifiers from data collection forms and computer files whenever feasible, and reinforcing the importance of maintaining the confidentiality of health records during orientation and training sessions for study personnel. Results should only be released in tabulated or aggregate form to prevent identification of individuals and breaches of confidentiality.

Many valid forms of research (e.g., pharmacoepidemiology, outcomes research, health services research utilizing health claims data, etc.) require access to personal information in databases assembled and maintained for purposes other than health research. For the public to derive benefits from research studies using health claims data, some minor incursions of privacy by qualified health researchers are deemed permissible. Social benefits of such studies include the identification of disease-risk factor associations, cost-benefit analyses of health claims data, and studies of the quality and effectiveness of health care. Such studies can contribute to the formulation of sound health policy.

When researchers use large databases, their focus is on the estimation of overall measures of association and statistical analysis of aggregate data. With special safeguards such as approval by an independent review committee, researchers occasionally link information obtained from study participants to records maintained by outside agencies such as disease registries.

Potential risks from breaches of confidentiality must be minimized in such studies by strict adherence to confidentiality safeguards. It is generally impossible to obtain the informed consent of individuals whose health claims are included in such databases because of the vast numbers of records.

Studies made possible through the advent of powerful computers, which provide important information about the public's health, are of concern to some members of society who are especially sensitive to issues of privacy. Public health professionals must inform legislators (and the general public) about the social value of health research studies that use large databases, while respecting the opinions and perspectives of others who may hold dissenting viewpoints. Researchers who are privileged to have access to large databases for use in health research must rigorously protect the confidentiality of the information.

A number of ethical challenges posed by the need to protect privacy and confidentiality are illustrated in the cases that follow.

Case 2a: Ethical Dilemma Involving Confidentiality of Information Collected from Men at High Risk for HIV Infection

In an epidemiologic study of men at high risk for infection with the human immunodeficiency virus (HIV), confidentiality was promised to the participants regarding information collected in the study. The pledge was made by the researchers at the time the participants' informed consent was obtained. In the subsequently administered interview, the participants were asked whether they had donated blood during the past two years. Several participants who were found to be HIV antibody seropositive reported having given blood within the two years prior to the HIV antibody testing. It was not feasible to check whether or not the blood had been discarded by the Red Cross without breaching confidentiality and violating the researcher's pledge to the participants (Gordis, 1991).

Questions for Discussion

1.   How should the original commitment to the participants to maintain confidentiality be balanced against the need to determine whether anyone had received contaminated blood from these donors so that further transmission of HIV might be prevented?
2.   Do researchers have a responsibility to anticipate such dilemmas before obtaining the informed consent of the research participants?

Reference

Gordis, L. (1991). Ethical and professional issues in the changing practice of epidemiology. *J Clin Epidemiol*, 44,(Suppl. I), 9S-13S.

Case 2b: State Privacy Laws Governing Access to Medical Records as an Obstacle to Epidemiologic Research

Federal regulations and state laws protecting the confidentiality of health records and their interpretation by local institutional review boards (IRBs) sometimes pose barriers to legitimate hospital-based studies. In Louisiana, for example, strict interpretation of state privacy laws precludes epidemiologists from gaining access to medical records without first obtaining the consent of each patient. Only cancer registries and studies based upon vital statistics records are exempt.

In one instance, an IRB in New Orleans required investigators to adopt a protocol that would have the attending physician sign and forward a letter to the patients, informing them about the study and how to contact the researchers if they wanted to participate. The intent of this requirement was to bypass the privacy laws governing the release of hospital records and to prevent lawsuits by disgruntled patients who might become incensed by researchers gaining access to their records without their consent. This requirement, which contributes little to the protection of patient privacy beyond that afforded by existing safeguards, would diminish the response rate and diminish the scientific validity of the study, as well as prevent the patient from learning that the investigators had already reviewed their hospital records in order to identify eligible cases.

Questions for Discussion
1.   How should the need to respect the rights of patients to privacy be balanced against researchers' need for access to health records?
2.   Under what circumstances can researchers bypass the requirement that they obtain the informed consent of patients before gaining access to their medical records?
3.   What steps should researchers take to protect the confidentiality of health information collected in hospital-based studies?

Case 2c: Release of Cancer Registry Data to a Third Party
Coal tar left in partly destroyed underground tanks at a coal gasification plant in Taylorville, Illinois, was blamed for a number of cases of neuroblastoma in children who lived in the community. The children and their parents sued Central Illinois Public Service Company and an engineering firm. In 1992, the

Illinois Department of Public Health was served with a subpoena demanding that "files of the Division of Epidemiology and Division of Environmental Health" be turned over to the court. The director of the Illinois Department of Public Health was served a related subpoena in 1993 demanding an exhaustive list of documents relating to the department's neuroblastoma data.

The department and its officers responded by saying that the documents were privileged health data and that maintaining the confidentiality of the data was essential to the public's health. Public confidence that such data would be kept confidential was said to be vital for protecting the usefulness of the information.

A circuit court responded by ordering the department to produce the cancer registry by listing the type of cancer, date of diagnosis and zip code for each cancer patient. The department proposed substituting county for zip code, but this was rejected by the court. The state and the department sought to appeal the ruling, arguing that "the State of Illinois is filled with small communities, many with their own post offices. Approximately half of the incorporated cities and villages in this State have less than 1,000 people ... [given the release of the requested information] the ability to pinpoint a particular cancer victim is virtually assured."

Questions for Discussion

1   What rules should we have to help the appeals court address the confidentiality claim?
2.   How should confidentiality concerns be weighed against any rights the neuroblastoma victims might have to compensation?

Reference

May v. Central Illinois Public Service Co., 633 N.E.2d 97 (Ill. App.), pet. for appeal denied, 642 N.E.2d 1284 (Ill. 1984).

Suggestions for Further Reading

Annas, G. J. (1993). Privacy rules for DNA databanks: Protecting coded 'future diaries'. *JAMA*, 270, 2346-2350.
Applebaum, P. S., Roth, L. H. & Detre, T. (1984). Researchers' access to patient records: An analysis of the ethical problems. *Clin Res*, 32, 399-403.

Bayer, R., Levine, C. & Murray, T. H. (1984). Guidelines for confidentiality in research on AIDS. *IRB*, 6, 1-7.

Clarke, E. A., Darlington, G., Holowaty, E. J., et al. (1993). Confidentiality and research. *Canadian Med Assoc J*, 149, 792-3.

Curran, W. J. (1986). The Privacy Protection Report and epidemiological research. *Am J Public Health*, 68, 173.

Curran, W. J. (1986). Protecting confidentiality in epidemiologic investigations by the Centers for Disease Control. *N Engl J Med*, 314, 1027-1028.

Feinleib, M. (1991). The epidemiologist's responsibilities to study participants. *J Clin Epidemiol*, 44,(Suppl. I), 73S-79S.

Gordis, L. & Gold, E. (1980). Privacy, confidentiality, and the use of medical records in research. *Science*, 207, 153-156.

Gordis, L., Gold, E. & Seltser, R. (1977). Privacy protection in epidemiologic and medical research: A challenge and a responsibility. *Am J Epidemiol*, 105, 163-168.

Gold, E. (1996). Confidentiality and privacy protection in epidemiologic research. In S. S. Coughlin & T. L. Beauchamp (Eds.). *Ethics and epidemiology* (pp. 128-141). New York: Oxford University Press.

Gostin, L., Turek-Brezina, J., Powers, M., et al. (1993). Privacy and security of personal information in a new health care system. *J Am Med Assoc*, 270, 2487-2493.

Holder, A. R. (1986). The biomedical researcher and subpoenas: Judicial protection of confidential medical data. *Am J Law Med*, 12, 405-421.

James, R. C. (1996). Data protection and epidemiologic research. *Science of the Total Environment*, 184, 25-32.

Kelsey, J. L. (1981). Privacy and confidentiality in epidemiological research involving patients. *IRB*, 3, 1-4.

Lako, C. J. (1986). Privacy protection and population-based health research. *Soc Sci Med*, 23, 293-295.

Marwick, C. (1984). Epidemiologists strive to maintain confidentiality of some health data. *JAMA*, 252, 2377-2383.

McCarthy, C. R. & Porter, J. P. (1991). Confidentiality: The protection of personal data in epidemiological and clinical research trials. *Law Med Health Care*, 19,238-241.

National Center for Health Statistics. (1984). NCHS staff manual on confidentiality. Hyattsville, MD.

Nehls, G. J., Hayes, C. G. & Nelson, W. C. (1981). Confidentiality and freedom of information for epidemiological data in governmental research. *Environ Res*, 25, 160-166.

Privacy Protection Study Commission. (1977). Personal Privacy in an Information Society. Washington, DC: Government Printing Office.

Soskolne, C. L. (1975). Privacy and data banks. *Humanitas RSA*, 3, 37-45.

Torres, C. G., Turner, M. E., Harkess, J. R., et al. (1991). Security measures for AIDS and HIV. A*m J Public Health*, 81, 210-211.

Wallace, R. J. (1982). Privacy and the use of data in epidemiology. In T. L. Beauchamp, R. R. Faden, R. J. Wallace & L. Walters (Eds.). *Ethical issues in social science research*. Baltimore: The Johns Hopkins University Press.

Westrin, C. G. & Nilstun, T. (1994). The ethics of data utilization: a comparison between epidemiology and journalism. *BMJ*, 308, 522-523.

Chapter 3

Informed Consent in Public Health Research

Informed or valid consent has been a central part of biomedical ethics since the trials of Nazi physicians at Nuremberg. Virtually all codes of professional conduct for health professionals and researchers require that the informed consent of patients and study participants be obtained before any intervention or participation in research. Ongoing public health problems such as the AIDS epidemic have raised a number of important issues related to informed consent including whether information provided to participants in research studies is adequate and whether it is permissible to test for HIV antibody status without informing the patient or participant.

Informed consent provisions attempt to ensure that patients and research participants make free choices, and encourage health professionals to act responsibly in their interactions with patients. They also provide institutions with legally valid authorization to proceed with interventions or therapeutic procedures. In recent years, focus has been placed not only on the obligation of investigators to disclose information, but also on the quality of the understanding and consent of the patient or research participant.

The five individual elements of informed consent are competence, disclosure, understanding, voluntariness, and consent. As Beauchamp and Childress (1994) have explained, "One gives an informed consent to an intervention if one is competent to act, receives a thorough disclosure, comprehends the disclosure, acts voluntarily, and consents to the intervention." This five-element definition has advantages over earlier definitions involving disclosure that have stemmed from medical malpractice law.

Investigators are obligated to disclose those facts or descriptions that patients or other individuals usually consider salient in deciding whether to consent to a proposed intervention or therapeutic procedure. In the case of research studies and clinical trials, information must be provided about the purpose of the research, the scientific methods and procedures, any anticipated risks and benefits, any anticipated inconveniences or discomfort, and the individuals' right to refuse participation or to withdraw from the research at any time without penalty.

The adequacy of information disclosed to patients enrolled in clinical trials of experimental therapies has undergone scrutiny, along with the ability of research participants to comprehend the information presented about potential risks and benefits. Critics have charged that informed consent statements in such trials often are written in the style of a scientific article and may require the reading comprehension level of a college graduate.

There have been extended discussion and debate over the adequacy of provisions for obtaining the consent of participants in studies conducted in developing countries by investigators from the United States and Europe. For example, in randomized controlled trials of HIV vaccines in Africa, Asia, and South America, informed consent should be obtained from each individual participant, rather than exclusively from male heads-of-household or community leaders.

Instances of testing for HIV antibody status and other serologic markers without the knowledge or consent of patients and research participants have generated controversy. Ethical considerations and legal protections require that the informed consent of patients be obtained before they are tested for HIV status, even in situations where the welfare of health care workers or other third parties is of concern. An important exception is anonymous unlinked testing for HIV antibody in "seroprevalence" surveys conducted in the United States and some other countries.

Many of these issues surrounding informed consent in public health research are illustrated by the case studies provided in this chapter.

References

Beauchamp, T. L. & Childress, J. F. (1994). *Principles of biomedical ethics* (4th ed.). New York: Oxford University Press.

Faden, R. R. & Beauchamp, T. L. (1986). *A history and theory of informed consent.* New York: Oxford University Press.

Case 3a: Adequacy of Informed Consent in a Seroepidemiologic Study of HTLV-II in Panamanian Children

Researchers are interested in testing frozen sera obtained in a 1991 survey of 760 Panamanian children between the ages of 2 and 12 for antibodies to human T-cell lymphotrophic virus Type II (HTLV-II). The banked sera were obtained as part of an earlier epidemiologic study of *Toxoplasma gondii* conducted in 13 mainland and island communities in Panama, which are inhabited by Indians. Testing for HTLV-II was not envisioned at the time the sera were originally collected.

The epidemiology of HTLV-II remains poorly understood. Endemic foci of HTLV-II infection have been reported in American Indian populations in New Mexico, Florida, and Brazil. A high seroprevalence of HTLV-II has also been found in a separate group of Indians in Panama (who reside on the other side of the country from the surveyed children). HTLV-II infection is common among injecting drug users in the United States. HTLV-II can be transmitted sexually and by exposure to cellular blood products. The high prevalence of HTLV-II infection among injecting drug users is presumed to be from the sharing of contaminated needles. There is limited evidence of the vertical transmission of HTLV-II from mother to child in the presence or absence of breast feeding.

The risks associated with infection by HTLV-II are poorly defined. HTLV-II has been isolated from the transformed T cells of a patient with hairy-cell leukemia (HCL) and also from a patient with T-cell lymphoproliferative disease and B-cell HCL. However, HTLV-II infection is not seen in most HCL patients. HTLV-II infections also have been described in isolated patients with aplastic anemia and prolymphocytic leukemia. No malignancies or other human diseases have been consistently and convincingly associated with HTLV-II infection. An association between HTLV-II and chronic fatigue syndrome has been reported.

Questions for Discussion

1.   If the sera collected and stored in 1991 (as part of an unrelated study) are tested for HTLV-II, should each research participant's mother have the right to provide surrogate informed consent for her underage child?
2.   What information should be conveyed to the participants to ensure that their consent is truly informed?
3.   If it were not feasible to contact the participants to obtain some additional form of informed consent, would the seroprevalence study of banked frozen sera be ethical?
4.   Should representatives of the Indian communities be notified that the study is being undertaken? What obligations would the investigators have to notify the participants (or their parents) of their test results?
5.   What precautions should the investigators take to protect the individual participants or the Indian communities as a whole from possible discrimination or other adverse effects?

References

Coughlin, S. S. (in press). HTLV-I/II. In *Encyclopedia of AIDS. A social, political, cultural and scientific record of the epidemic.* New York: Garland Publishing Inc..

Hjelle, B. (1991). Human T-cell leukemia/lymphoma viruses. Life cycle, pathogenicity, epidemiology, and diagnosis. *Arch Pathol Lab Med,* 115, 440-450.

Case 3b: Intentional Nondisclosure of Information in a Study of Cocaine Use Among Minority Inner-City Clinic Patients

Controversy arose over a study of the prevalence of cocaine use among low-income, predominantly African American patients seen at an inner-city hospital clinic. An important goal of the study, which was approved by an institutional review board, was to determine the validity of self-reported cocaine use in this population.

The researchers asked clinic patients to participate in a study of sexually transmitted diseases (STDs) in return for an incentive of ten dollars. Informed consent was obtained from the participants for the study of STDs, but not for the undisclosed study of the prevalence of cocaine use and the validity of self-reported information about cocaine use. The participants were told that their urine would be tested for STDs, but were unaware that it also would be tested for cocaine metabolites.

The response rate among eligible patients was 82 percent. The participants averaged about 30 years of age. About 92 percent were African Americans and 89 percent were uninsured. Among male participants, 39 percent (162 of 415) tested positive for a major cocaine metabolite in their urine. Among those with positive urine tests, however, 72 percent denied any illicit drug use in the recent past.

Questions for Discussion

1.   What was the ethical challenge faced by these investigators in their attempt to obtain accurate information about cocaine use and the reliability of patient self-reports? If they had been fully informed about the objectives of the study, how would many of the potential participants probably have responded?

2.   How does the fact that this study dealt with illicit drug use bear on the ethical analysis of this case?

3.   Under what circumstances, if any, is intentional nondisclosure of information permissible in research studies?

4.   What information should normally be disclosed to potential participants in research studies when their informed consent is obtained?

References

Beauchamp, T. L. & Childress, J. F. (1994). *Principles of biomedical ethics*, (4th ed.). New York: Oxford University Press.

McNagy, S. E. & Parker, R. M. (1992). High prevalence of recent cocaine use and the unreliability of patient self-report in an inner-city walk-in clinic. *JAMA*, 167, 1106-1108.

Case 3c: Duty to Inform Participants in United States Government-Sponsored Radiation Experiments

In the 1940s, several cancer patients, mostly civilians, were injected with radioactive thorotrast in a range of doses, without their knowledge or consent. The purpose of the experiments, which were conducted in hospitals in North America and Europe, was to determine the effect of radioactive explosion fallout on human populations. Although most of the patients who were injected died with malignant tumors within 18 months, there were some survivors.

By 1960, a longitudinal study of the survivors had been undertaken by an international research team of university and government scientists to determine the long-term effects of radioactive contamination on the human body. The study included a cohort of survivors and controls who had had no exposure to radioactive thorotrast. From 1960 to 1978, the research team found a significantly higher number of malignancies in the experimental group than in the control group. The participants were not informed about their injections because it was believed that nothing could be done in addition to monitoring them, which was already being done. There was also concern about needlessly alarming them. The physicians who examined the surviving participants were informed about the radiation exposures.

Questions for Discussion

1.   Whose interests were served by the decision not to tell the participants that they had been injected with radioactive material?
2.   Should the participants have been informed of their radiation exposure even though they might have been alarmed by this disclosure?
3.   Is research on people without their informed consent ever permissible, as in the interests of "national security" or in time of war?
4.   Should the governments that sponsored the experiments be expected to make financial compensation to the survivors or their next of kin?

Suggestions for Further Reading

Advisory Committee on Human Radiation Experiments. (1996). *The human radiation experiments: Final report of the president's advisory committee.* New York: Oxford University Press.

Annas, G. J. (1996). Questing for grails: Duplicity, betrayal and self-deception in postmodern medical research. *J Contemp Health Law Pol, 12,* 297-324.

Coughlin, S. S. (in press). Informed consent. In *Encyclopedia of AIDS. A social, political, cultural and scientific record of the epidemic.* New York: Garland Publishing, Inc.

Fletcher, J. C., (1983). The evolution of the ethics of informed consent. In K. Berg & K. E. Trany (Eds.),*Research Ethics.* (pp. 187-228). New York: Alan R. Liss, Inc.

Makarushka, J. & McDonald, R. (1979). Informed consent, research, and geriatric patients: The responsibility of institutional review committees. *The Gerontologist, 19,* 61-66.

Schulte, P. A. & Singal, M. (1996). Ethical issues in the interaction with subjects and disclosure of results. In S. S. Coughlin & T. L. Beauchamp (Eds.). *Ethics and epidemiology* (pp. 178-96). New York: Oxford University Press.

Shultz, M. M. (1996). Legal and ethical considerations for securing consent to epidemiologic research in the United States. In S. S. Coughlin & T. L. Beauchamp (Eds.). *Ethics and epidemiology.* (pp. 97-127). New York: Oxford University Press.

Taub, H. (1986). Comprehension of informed consent for research: Issues and directions for future study. *IRB, 8,* 7-10.

Taub, H., Baker, M. & Sturr, J. (1986). Informed consent for research: effects of readability, patient age, and education. *J Am Geriatrics Soc, 34,* 601-606.

Warren, J., Sobal, J., Tenney, J., et al. (1986). Informed consent by proxy. *N Engl J Med, 315,* 1124-1128.

Chapter 4

Randomized Controlled Trials

S ince the late 1940s, when the Medical Research Council Streptomycin in Tuberculosis Trial was undertaken, the randomized controlled trial has become a preferred means of evaluating clinical therapies. The enhanced scientific validity of this method is partly attributable to the randomization process, which tends to produce treatment and control groups that are evenly balanced with respect to prognostic or confounding factors. With the use of alternative methods such as observational study designs or studies that rely on historical controls (in which all patients under investigation receive the new treatment), the treatment and control groups are less likely to be comparable. The large-scale use of randomized controlled trials in recent decades has revolutionized clinical investigation and the manner in which new therapies are introduced.

There has been ongoing debate over the ethics of randomized controlled trials, which frequently require the balancing of potential benefits to individual patients against those that may be gained by future patients, or society. A tension may exist in clinical trials between the physician's or nurse's responsibility to act in the best interest of individual patients and the societal need to acquire new knowledge by randomizing patients to therapy according to a standard protocol. Many argue that for randomized controlled trials to be ethical, there must be genuine uncertainty about the comparative therapeutic merits of each treatment arm; that is, a state of *equipoise* must exit. It is unethical to withhold a beneficial treatment unless there is good reason to believe that the new treatment will be at least as effective. The control treatment ought to consist of the best available standard treatment of the disease under study. When a new treatment is known to be superior to alternative treatments, then randomization is unnecessary and should not be undertaken. The use of placebo controls may be ethically permissible as long as no therapy of proven value exists and the informed consent of the participants is obtained. The use of placebo controls is generally proscribed when there is a standard therapy of proven value.

A data-monitoring committee is commonly employed to review the evidence emerging from a clinical trial and to stop the trial when there is decisive evidence in favor of one treatment. However, as Tagnon (1984) has argued, investigators have an ethical obligation to avoid stopping trials of experimental therapies prematurely before a firm conclusion has been reached. Prematurely stopping a trial may "lead to new trials and the involvement of more patients receiving an untested treatment." (Tagnon, 1984: 19). Ethically optimized clinical trial designs have been proposed, including adaptive and sequential designs that ensure that the fewest possible number of patients receive the less effective therapy. Such designs have not been widely used, however, and are not always ethically or statistically defensible.

A number of ethical issues arising in randomized controlled trials are highlighted in the cases presented in this chapter.

References

Coughlin, S. S. (Ed.). (1995). *Ethics in epidemiology and clinical research: Annotated readings.* Chestnut Hill, MA: Epidemiology Resources Inc.

Hellman, S. & Hellman, D. S. (1991). Of mice but not men. Problems of the randomized clinical trial. *N Engl J Med, 324,* 1585-1589.

Soskolne, C. L. & MacFarlane, D. K. (1996). Scientific misconduct in epidemiologic research. In S. S. Coughlin & T. L. Beauchamp (Eds.). *Ethics and epidemiology.* (pp. 274-289). New York: Oxford University Press.

Tagnon, H. J. (1984). Ethical considerations in controlled clinical trials. In M. E. Buyse, M. J. Staquet & R. J. Sylvester (Eds.). *Cancer clinical trials. Methods and practice* (pp. 14-25). New York: Oxford University Press.

Case 4a: Randomized Controlled Trials of Bone Marrow Transplants for the Treatment of Advanced Breast Cancer in Women

An increasing number of women with advanced breast cancer are convinced that a bone marrow transplant, which involves a very high dose of chemotherapy followed by the transplant, is the best treatment option. In many cases, their doctors agree. The effectiveness of this treatment for advanced breast cancer has not been conclusively demonstrated, however.

The National Cancer Institute in the United States is sponsoring three large randomized trials to determine whether bone marrow transplants are preferable to the chemotherapy regimens that are now standard treatment for advanced breast cancer. In these trials, about half of the participants are randomly allocated to receive the transplant and the balance receive the standard treatment. Many women with advanced breast cancer are turning to bone marrow transplants outside of scientific trials, however. In view of poor survival rates associated with conventional treatments, they are unwilling to take the chance they will not be assigned to the experimental group. As a result, researchers are having difficulty enrolling enough participants in the trials. Without proper studies, there is a danger that no one will ever know whether the transplants are actually preferable to conventional treatments.

The transplants are grueling and risky for the breast cancer patients. Roughly 5 percent of women who undergo a bone marrow transplant die as a result of the treatment. The transplants are also expensive. Whereas conventional chemotherapy costs $5,000 to $25,000, bone marrow transplants run from $60,000 to $200,000. In response to lawsuits, an increasing number of insurance companies have agreed to pay for the transplants.

Questions for Discussion

1.   In 1994 alone, more than 1,000 women with breast cancer underwent bone marrow transplants in the United States outside of clinical trials. Would it be ethical to require patients to enroll in a clinical trial in order to gain access to this experimental therapy?

2.   What would be the risks and potential benefits if this expensive new treatment were to become the treatment-of-choice for advanced breast cancer, with or without adequate evidence from randomized clinical trials?

3.   Is it ethical for a physician investigator to enroll his or her patients in a randomized trial of bone marrow transplants if he/she is fairly sure, but not absolutely sure, that the transplants are better than conventional therapy?

4.   Clinical researchers often have a stake in the timely completion of clinical trials. In those situations where physicians have a financial or professional incentive to maximize the number of their patients enrolled in a trial, to what extent does this represent conflicting interests?

Reference

Women rejecting trials for testing a cancer therapy. (1995, February 15). *The New York Times.*

Case 4b: Randomized Controlled Trial of Continuous Oxygen Administration in Premature Infants at Risk for Retrolental Fibroplasia

The epidemic of blindness from retrolental fibroplasia arose abruptly in the 1940s, primarily among premature infants. Of the more than 50 causes of retrolental fibroplasia proposed at that time, only four were examined using randomized trials. Based upon observational evidence, attention gradually focused on the oxygen-rich environment that was routinely provided to premature babies. There was intense scientific debate in the 1950s over whether oxygen was the causative factor. At a meeting called by the National Institutes of Health in 1953, most of the scientists present believed that a multicenter clinical trial should be conducted to examine this question. Some of those in attendance, however, believed that there was already enough evidence from observational studies and opposed the trial on ethical grounds.

The trial was initiated in July 1953. Almost 800 infants were studied at 18 participating hospitals. Retrolental fibroplasia occurred in 23 percent of the infants who received oxygen routinely as compared with only 7 percent of those who received reduced oxygen. The release of these dramatic results in 1954 quickly led to the widespread modification of the practice of routinely exposing premature infants to an oxygen-rich environment. The epidemic of this form of blindness, which had ironically resulted from the well-intentioned efforts of physicians to increase the survival of premature babies, quickly subsided.

Questions for Discussion

1.   Is it ethical for investigators to conduct a randomized clinical trial if they are fairly certain, on the basis of nonexperimental evidence, that patients enrolled in one treatment arm or the other will experience significant side effects? What if the expected side effects are severe or irreversible, as in the case of blindness from retrolental fibroplasia?
2.   What are the potential risks of not having conclusive evidence from randomized clinical trials?

Reference

Silverman, W. A. (1977). The lesson of retrolental fibroplasia. *Scientific American*, 236, 100-107.

Case 4c: Trial of Tamoxifen in the Primary Prevention of Breast Cancer

(This case study, which was written by Douglas Weed and Steven Coughlin, is reprinted by permission of Marcel-Dekker, Inc.)

A randomized controlled trial of tamoxifen as a chemopreventive agent in postmenopausal women at increased risk of breast cancer has been undertaken and has accrued over half of the study population required. Although the women who are enrolled in the trial may have a pronounced family history of breast cancer, they are generally asymptomatic or free of disease at baseline, and they may not develop breast cancer even in the absence of any preventive therapy. Thus, healthy individuals are randomly allocated to receive either tamoxifen or placebo, and they will be exposed to this hormonal agent over several years.

The trial will require large numbers of individuals (approximately 16,000) and large amounts of funding and other resources.

Although the efficacy of tamoxifen as a chemopreventive agent remains unproven, the potential benefits of tamoxifen to the individual research participants and to society are substantial. Breast cancer is the second leading cause of cancer death among women in the United States, and one in nine women may develop breast cancer in her lifetime—although this number has been both misunderstood and recently revised. Breast cancer is arguably one of the most important health concerns among women and provides an important context for the estimation that tamoxifen intervention could reduce breast cancer risk by as much as 50 percent. Toxicity trials have suggested that tamoxifen also may have beneficial effects on blood lipids that predispose individuals to coronary atherosclerosis. For example, one controlled trial involving 140 postmenopausal women with axillary node-negative breast cancer (Love et al., 1990) demonstrated that a standard regimen of tamoxifen reduced total blood cholesterol by an average of 20 percent. Tamoxifen therapy also may reduce the morbidity associated with osteoporosis.

The potential side effects of tamoxifen are only partially understood. Long-term tamoxifen therapy has been associated with pulmonary embolism and other thromboembolic conditions. In addition, tamoxifen has been associated with an increased risk of endometrial cancer. Women treated with tamoxifen also may be more likely to experience hot flashes, vaginitis, depression, and ocular changes such as macular edema, optic neuritis, and corneal changes. In addition, there may be side effects associated with long-term tamoxifen therapy that have not been identified by studies carried out to date.

Questions for Discussion

1.   What ethical issues must the investigators take into account in planning this trial?

2.   Is it ethical to expose participants to a chemopreventive agent that may have unexpected side effects or be ineffective? Conversely, are the potential risks outweighed by the potential benefits to the participants and to society?

3. How is this balancing of risks and potential benefits influenced by the choice of a study population?

4. Is it ethical for the investigators to deny possible benefits from the trial to women randomly allocated to the placebo group? Do the investigators have an ethical obligation to provide tamoxifen to high-risk women randomly allocated to the control group even though its effectiveness in chemoprevention has yet to be demonstrated?

5. What are the consequences of not conducting a trial of this nature among women at high risk for breast cancer?

6. Will the potential benefits and burdens of the trial be distributed equitably among the participants?

7. With respect to informed consent, to what extent are lay persons included in the trial likely to adequately understand the potential risks and benefits associated with participation in the trial?

References

Weed, D. L. & Coughlin, S. S. (1995). Ethics in cancer prevention and control. In P. Greenwald, B. F. Kramer & D. L. Weed (Eds.). *Cancer prevention and control*, (pp. 497-507). New York: Marcel-Dekker.

Love, R. R., Newcomb, P. A. & Wiebe, D. A. (1990). Lipid and lipoprotein effects of tamoxifen therapy in postmenopausal patients with node-negative breast cancer. *J Natl Cancer Inst, 82,* 1327-1332.

Nayfield, S. G., Karp, J. E. & Ford, L. G. (1991). Potential role of tamoxifen in prevention of breast cancer. *J Natl Cancer Inst, 83,* 1450-1490.

Suggestions for Further Reading

Freedman, B. (1987). Equipoise and the ethics of clinical research. *N Engl J Med, 317,* 141-145.

Howard-Jones, N. (1982). Human experimentation in historical and ethical perspectives. *Soc Sci Med, 16,* 1429-1448.

Johnson, N., Lilford, R. J. & Brazier, W. (1991). At what level of collective equipoise does a clinical trial become ethical? *J Med Ethics, 17,* 30-34.

Levine, C. (1988). Has AIDS changed the ethics of human subjects research? *IRB*, 16, 167-173.

Levine, R. J. (1985). The use of placebos in randomized clinical trials. *IRB*, 7, 1.

Levine, R. J. (1991). Comment re: "Ethics and statistics in randomized clinical trials." *Stat Sci*, 6, 71-74.

Levine, R. J. The impact of HIV infection on society's perception of clinical trials. *Kennedy Inst Ethics J*, 4, 93-98.

Levine, R. J. & Lebacqz, K. (1979). Some ethical considerations in clinical trials. *Clin Pharm Ther*, 25, 728-741.

Macklin, R. & Friedland, G. (1986). AIDS Research: The ethics of clinical trials. *Law Med Health Care*, 14, 273-280.

Passamani, E. (1991). Clinical trials—Are they ethical? *N Engl J Med*, 324, 1589-1592.

Rothman, K. J. & Michels, K. B. (1994). The continuing unethical use of placebo controls. *N Engl J Med*, 331, 394-398.

Royall, R. M. (1991). Ethics and statistics in randomized clinical trials. *Stat Sci*, 6, 52-88.

Taylor, K., Margolese, R. & Soskolne, C. L. (1984). Physicians' reasons for not entering eligible patients in a randomized clinical trial of surgery for breast cancer. *N Engl J Med*, 310, 1363-1367.

Weinstein, M. C. (1974). Allocation of subjects in medical experiments. *N Engl J Med*, 291, 1278-1285.

Zelen, M. (1991). Comment: The ethics of clinical trials. *Stat Sci*, 6, 81-83.

Chapter 5

Committee Review and the Institutional Review Board System

The ethics review of research protocols by an independent committee ensures that the rights and welfare of study participants are protected and that the potential benefits outweigh the risks to participants (where this is appropriate). Before embarking on a study, researchers are obligated by law to submit a protocol describing the study methods and its significance to a review committee known in the United States as an institutional review board (IRB). Committee members, including professionals and lay persons, must be independent from the investigators and the research sponsor or funding agency.

In addition to reviewing the research protocol, members of review committees should carefully examine the informed consent statement submitted by the investigators for its completeness and clarity. Provisions for obtaining the informed consent of participants respect their autonomous right to make informed decisions about whether to participate in the study (as discussed in Chapter 3). Consent statements must be written in language that is understandable to a lay person. The members of the review committee also should ensure that there is no manipulation or coercion in recruiting research participants.

Adequate precautions must be taken by investigators to minimize risks or potential harms. Studies that provide benefits to society, but not to the research participants themselves, may be acceptable as long as the risks to participants are minor and they are informed of these risks and potential benefits.

In addition to minimizing risks and ensuring the safety of the study participants, researchers are also responsible for the safety of the study team.

Even if great care has been taken in developing a study protocol that minimizes risks, maximizes potential benefits, and adequately informs the research participants, the investigators' ethical and professional obligations are far from over. Ethical considerations arise in every phase of studies, from their initial design to the publication and dissemination of the final results.

A number of ethical issues related to committee review and the IRB system in the United States are highlighted in the case studies that follow.

Case 5a: Multi-Institutional Review of a Research Protocol as a Barrier to Human Subjects Research

Investigators planned a multicenter study of genetic counseling services and began seeking approval from IRBs at 51 institutions in 1976 (Kavanagh et al., 1979). Their study, which was funded by the National Foundation—March of Dimes, was designed to provide data on the organization, operation, and effectiveness of genetic counseling. The data were to be collected from providers and clients.

After the protocol was approved by the IRB at their home institution, the investigators contacted clinic directors at institutions receiving National Foundation grants for genetic counseling services and sought their participation. Fifty-one of the clinic directors agreed to participate in the study; they were asked to act as the investigators' intermediaries in seeking IRB approval at the local institutions.

Eleven of the centers informed the investigators that no IRB review was needed at their institutions. At 28 institutions, the IRB approved the protocol without revisions; approval at these institutions required 146 telephone calls and 49 letters on the part of the investigators. Twelve IRBs approved the protocol after requesting at least one revision; most of the required revisions related to the informed consent form. Final approval at these 12 institutions required 96 telephone calls and 41 letters. One institution refused to review the protocol because "only two of [their] doctors were involved in the study. ..."

On the basis of their frustrating and time-consuming experience, the investigators argued for the development of "more uniform, clearly defined review policies, including clearer provisions for social science research, and more expeditious procedures for multi-institutional review." (p. 3).

Questions for Discussion

1.   What is the purpose of committee reviews like that conducted by IRBs in the United States? In what ways do IRBs protect the rights and welfare of research participants?

2.   To what extent do IRBs protect the interests of their own institutions as opposed to those of research participants?

3.   Should local committees review research protocols throughout the United States and other countries, or should national review committees be set up?

4.   How can the needs of multicenter research studies and clinical trials be accommodated? Should there be a single informed consent statement in such studies, or should these be revised in accordance with the requirements of each participating center?

Reference

Kavanagh, C., Matthews, D., Sorenson, J. R. & Swazey, J. P. (1979). We shall overcome: Multi-institutional review of a genetic counseling study. *IRB*, 1, 1-3.

Case 5b: Institutional Review Board Concern Over a Retrospective Study of Clinical Test Results

A study was planned by government researchers in the United States to examine the sensitivity and specificity of a particular diagnostic test. The project involved retrospectively accessing a clinical database to identify test results for persons who had undergone a battery of tests. The investigators planned to interview the patients identified in this way to obtain further information. At the time the battery of tests had been completed, the implications of a positive result for the test of interest (in terms of clinical significance or personal decision making) were unclear.

IRB members who reviewed the study protocol were concerned that the investigators intended to contact the patients without first contacting their family doctors or primary care physicians. They were afraid that the patients would object to this breach of confidentiality and unauthorized release of personal medical information, and that complaints and possible litigation could arise. It was unlikely that the physicians had followed-up on positive results or discussed such results with their patients, since the battery of tests was difficult to interpret and the implications of a positive test result were unclear at the time of completion.

The members of the IRB attempted to avoid potential conflicts by requiring the investigators to notify the physicians that they were interested in contacting their patients to invite them to participate in the study, and to obtain the assent of each patient's physician. This provided the physicians some measure of control over which patients would be contacted for the purposes of this research study.

Questions for Discussion

1.   Did the IRB arrive at a satisfactory resolution to this confidentiality problem? Should each patient's physician be consulted in situations such as this one, to determine whether it is "medically advisable" for the patient to be contacted and invited to take part in a research study?

2.   What types of policies would be helpful in governing the retrospective use of clinical records for the purposes of health research?

3.   What additional safeguards are needed in those situations in which it is necessary to contact former patients for some additional form of research?

Case 5c: IRB Review of a Needle Exchange Program Evaluation Study

Needle exchange programs, in which intravenous drug users trade used needles for free, sterile ones, are generally thought to reduce the spread of HIV infection, hepatitis, and other blood-borne contagious conditions. It is possible, however, that part of the success of such programs is the result of self-selection by drug users who are already inclined to repair their lives and are more likely to participate in the exchange program.

To examine these issues, a study was proposed that would randomize 600 intravenous drug users into two groups: one group could exchange used needles for sterile ones; the other group could not, but would be told where to acquire clean needles inexpensively and legally. All participants would be referred to treatment programs if desired.

The protocol was approved by a local IRB and by the federal Office of Protection from Research Risks. Nevertheless, the proposed study has generated considerable controversy.

Opponents of the study contend that it would unnecessarily expose members of the second group to increased risk of disease and constitute the withholding of a lifesaving device. Others argue that careful studies are still needed to acquire important data about the self-selection hypothesis and that the availability of cheap needles and treatment programs for the second group would reduce their risk to acceptable levels.

Questions for Discussion

1.   Suppose an IRB of which you were a member was evaluating this study: What position would you take, and why?
2.   Assume that members of the second group would, in fact, face an increased risk of disease. Does the information that would be gained by this study provide sufficient justification for placing individuals at increased risk of serious disease? Does it matter that all of the participants will have given their informed consent?
3.   Although several observational (nonrandomized) studies have already shown the utility of needle exchange programs, the United States Government does not provide funding for such programs, which are politically controversial. How much financial support should be provided for evaluating controversial public health programs such as needle exchange programs, condom giveaways, and so forth?

Reference

Schartz, J. (1996, October 18). NIH to review needle exchange study criticized for possible medical risk. *The Washington Post*, p. A25.

Suggestions for Further Reading

Cann, C. I. & Rothman, K. J. (1984). IRBs and epidemiologic research: How inappropriate restrictions hamper studies. *IRB*, 6, 5-7.

Greenwald, R. A., Ryan, M. K. & Mulvihill, J.E., (Eds.). (1982). *Human subjects research: A handbook for institutional review boards*. New York: Plenum Press.

Levine, R. J. (1996). The institutional review board. In S. S. Coughlin & T. L. Beauchamp (Eds.). *Ethics and epidemiology*, (pp. 257-273). New York: Oxford University Press.

Levine, R. J. (1986). *Ethics and regulation of clinical research*. New Haven: Yale University Press.

Macrina, F. L. (1995). *Scientific integrity. An introductory text with cases*. Washington, DC: American Society for Microbiology.

McNeill, P. M. (1989). Research ethics committees in Australia, Europe, and North America. *IRB*, 11, 4-7.

Office for Protection from Research Risks. (1993). Protecting human research subjects: Institutional review board guidebook. Washington, DC: U.S. Government Printing Office.

Robertson, J. A. (1982). Taking consent seriously: IRB intervention in the consent process. *IRB*, 4, 1-5.

Robertson, J. A. (1979). The law of institutional review boards. *UCLA Law Rev*, 26, 484-549.

Robertson, J. A. (1979). Ten ways to improve IRBs. *Hastings Center Rep*, 9, 29-33.

Williams, P. C. (1984). Success in spite of failure: Why IRBs falter in reviewing risks and benefits. *IRB*, 6, 1-4.

Chapter 6

Scientific Misconduct in Public Health Research

M any people believe that those following careers in any of the health sciences are virtuous and trustworthy, protect the public interest, and possess a desire to pursue truth. This belief, however, does not always reflect reality. Theft of intellectual property, plagiarism, and fabrication or falsification of data are all known to occur. Such practices fall under the general rubric of scientific misconduct (Soskolne & Macfarlane, 1996).

Besides damaging the pursuit of truth and the protection of the public interest, scientific misconduct has a further dimension. It affects the various aspects of interpersonal conduct not only among scientists, but also between scientists and the various constituency groups with whom public health researchers work. Two moral foundations upon which good collegial relationships rest are those of integrity and mutual trust, which, when eroded, severely damage relationships between colleagues.

Overzealousness also may drive misconduct. This can occur when the excitement that the researcher feels over his or her research leads to behaviors that are, at best, lacking in objectivity or, at worst, irrationally biased. In these circumstances, the necessary objectivity of the scientist is lost.

Those who make allegations of research misconduct—"whistleblowers"—may fear job loss or some form of retaliation, especially if those accused are in positions of authority over those making the allegations.

Guidelines for the handling of allegations of misconduct have been difficult to manage, and the issue of due process has become preeminent in investigations of this nature. Because allegations do not always prove to be true, the reputation of the accused should be protected unless guilt is established.

In the United States, the Office of Research Integrity (ORI) evolved within the U.S. Department of Health and Human Services (DHHS) in response to several highly publicized cases of scientific misconduct in the late 1970s. The authority of ORI to make findings of scientific misconduct and to propose Public Health Service administrative actions is founded in statute and regulation. The purpose of ORI is to protect the research mission of the Public Health Service.

Scientific misconduct can have an extremely negative impact on the public's perception of the scientific enterprise. This, in turn, can affect the allocation of public resources for science. In addition, scientific misconduct can impede the pursuit of truth, leading scientific inquiry in wasteful directions and squandering scarce resources.

The cases that follow illustrate several issues surrounding scientific misconduct, including the need for due process when allegations of misconduct are investigated.

References

Pellegrino, E. D. (1992). Character and the ethical conduct of research. *Accountability in research, 2,* 1-11.

Soskolne, C. L. & Macfarlane, D. K. (1996). Scientific misconduct in epidemiologic research. In S. S. Coughlin & T. L. Beauchamp (Eds), *Ethics and epidemiology* (pp. 274-289). New York: Oxford University Press.

Case 6a: *Removal of Bernard Fisher as Principal Investigator of the National Surgical Adjuvant Breast and Bowel Project*

The U.S. National Institutes of Health (NIH) called for Bernard Fisher to be replaced as the principal investigator of the National Surgical Adjuvant Breast and Bowel Project (NSABP) after it was determined that one of his co-investigators had falsified data on women who had entered a landmark multicenter clinical trial. The trial had shown that mastectomy conferred no advantage in survival over lumpectomy in women with breast cancer. The falsified data (from one cooperating center) consisted primarily of dates altered to make female patients eligible for the trial. Almost 500 cooperating centers were included in the trial.

This high-profile case of scientific misconduct received widespread coverage in the media. Women with breast cancer expressed anxiety over treatment decisions and shaken confidence in the reliability of medical research.

The allegations against Fisher related to the timing of reports disclosing the fact that data falsification had occurred in the trial. Fisher himself had not falsified any data and his group at the University of Pittsburgh was the first to question the data submitted to them from the cooperating center.

The NIH decision to remove Fisher raised questions in the minds of some epidemiologists and clinical trials researchers about whether Fisher was being scapegoated. The *Epidemiology Monitor* reported at the time, "'This investigator has won every kind of award known to humankind'—that's how one epidemiologist puzzled over the recent news that NIH was calling for the removal of Bernard Fisher" (p. 1).

In 1997, after nearly three years of investigation, the U.S. Department of Health and Human Services Office of Research Integrity (ORI) dismissed all scientific misconduct charges against Fisher.

Questions for Discussion

1.   What protections should investigators have against being penalized unjustly by funding agencies and other stakeholders for alleged improprieties—especially when the media and the public become involved?

2.   What responsibilities do investigators have for auditing and quality control of data collected by collaborators and co-investigators? To what lengths must researchers at coordinating centers go to verify data submitted to them from cooperating centers?

3.   What are the responsibilities of clinical trials researchers to the public, to funding agencies, and to their colleagues?

4.   To what extent do incidents of scientific misconduct damage the entire scientific enterprise through the erosion of public confidence and support?

References

NIH actions against breast cancer researcher raise issues for epidemiologists. (1994). *Epidemiology Monitor*, 15, 1-2.

Soskolne, C. L. & Macfarlane, D. K. (1996). Scientific misconduct in epidemiologic research. In S. S. Coughlin & T. L. Beauchamp (Eds.). *Ethics and epidemiology*. (pp. 274-289). New York: Oxford University Press.

Case 6b: Alleged Scientific Misconduct

A highly publicized case of alleged scientific misconduct was brought to light in 1992. The allegations revolved around the methods of analysis in pioneering work done in the 1970s on the neurobehavioral effects of environmental lead exposure in children. The controversy surfaced in 1992 and was widely covered by the media, even though the data in question had been reanalyzed several years previously. The investigator's name was ultimately cleared and this case of alleged scientific misconduct was dismissed.

Critics charged that the allegations were motivated by self-interest on the part of the lead industry. Many also felt that the investigation should have been kept confidential while it was ongoing. Such doubts raised concern among environmental scientists, government officials, and the general public. Considerable time, effort, and money were expended both by the investigator against whom the allegations were made and by those who investigated those allegations.

Questions for Discussion

1.   Should investigations into alleged cases of scientific misconduct be carried out in secrecy so as to protect the accused investigator from untoward publicity? What are the rights of individuals accused of scientific misconduct while the investigation is still ongoing, in terms of confidentiality and due process?

2.   To what extent are the scientific enterprise and society's interests protected by investigations into possible cases of scientific misconduct?

References

Soskolne, C. L. & Macfarlane, D. K. (1996). Scientific misconduct in epidemiologic research. In S. S. Coughlin & T. L. Beauchamp (Eds.). *Ethics and epidemiology.* (pp. 274-289). New York: Oxford University Press.

Wohleber, C. (1992, January 9). OSI asks for internal inquiry. Needleman challenged again on landmark 1979 study of low-lead exposure's effects, *University Times,* p. 4.

Case 6c: Possible Violation of Professional Standards by an Environmental Scientist

In a study funded and conducted jointly by a government and a university, a question arose over the dissemination of possibly misleading statements by a member of the research team. The team, composed of medical personnel, chemical and environmental experts, and health administrators, had been assembled to study possible chemical poisoning in a river basin near a large hydroelectric dam. Evidence of such environmental poisoning was, in fact, found. The medical experts proceeded to examine morbidity and mortality rates associated with the environmental contamination. The chemical and environmental experts began to assess the causes of and possible solutions to the pollution. The health administrators were charged with assessing the public health risk and determining the appropriate government response.

When an environmental expert began providing information to the news media, concern arose among the medical experts that she was greatly overstating the extent of the pollution problem. They charged that the expert was speaking outside of her area of expertise and exaggerating the health risks associated with the contamination. When the medical personnel began releasing reports that questioned the judgment of their collaborator, the integrity of the whole research project was called into question.

The critics among the medical personnel charged that the environmental expert was interested in attracting media attention to bring public attention to the issue before the research was concluded. They contended that she had an overly zealous, predetermined agenda and lacked scientific objectivity. On the other hand, the environmental expert believed that the team had gathered enough evidence to justify her statements to the media, and that it was her duty to act as an advocate for the victims of the chemical poisoning.

Questions for Discussion

1.   What are the obligations of health researchers to other members of their team in situations such as this? How can such conflicts between members of a research team be avoided?
2.   To what extent do incidents such as this lead to a lack of public trust in the whole scientific enterprise? What can the scientific community do to prevent such problems?
3.   Could the gender of the environmental expert have played a role in the criticisms expressed by other members of the research team against her?

Case 6d: Falsification of Data from an Environmental Study

An environmental study was undertaken because of concern over a spill of benzene-contaminated gasoline at an industrial site and a possible relationship between the spill and an increase in cancer rates in a nearby community. The study was conducted jointly by a research team from an area university and a team from the local hospital. One of the investigators at the hospital changed some data points in his portion of the project, rendering what would otherwise have been only slightly elevated risks into significantly elevated risks. His motivation may have been to make the results more sensational or to increase the likelihood of additional funding. The data falsification was subsequently brought to light after the results were submitted for publication in a peer-reviewed journal.

Questions for Discussion

1.   What precautions should scientists take in seeking out collaborators for interdisciplinary research projects?

2.   How can members of collaborative research groups guard against falsified or fabricated data?

3.   What are the obligations of researchers to society, to the profession, and to other members of the research group in a situation such as this one?

Suggestions for Further Reading

Broad, W. & Wade, N. (1982). *Betrayers of the truth: Fraud and deceit in the halls of science.* Simon and Schuster, New York.

Buzzelli, D. E. (1993). A definition of misconduct in science: A view from NSF. *Science,* 259, 584-585.

Caelleigh, A. S. (1993). Role of the journal editor in sustaining integrity in research. *Acad Med,* 68(Suppl.), S23-S29.

Goodstein, D. (1991). Scientific fraud. *Am Scholar,* 60, 505-515.

Knight, J. (1991). Scientific misconduct: The rights of the accused. *Issues in Science and Technology,* 8, 28-29.

Korenman, S. G. & Shipp, A. C. (1994). *Teaching the responsible conduct of research through a case study approach. A handbook for instructors.* Washington, DC: Association of American Medical Colleges.

Macrina, F. L. (1995). *Scientific integrity. An introductory text with cases.* Washington, DC: American Society for Microbiology.

Miller, D. J. & Hersen, M. (Eds.). (1992). *Research fraud in the behavioral and biomedical sciences.* New York: John Wiley & Sons, Inc.

Mishkin, B. (1988). Responding to scientific misconduct: Due process and prevention. *JAMA,* 260, 1932-1936.

National Academy of Sciences. (1992). *Responsible science: Ensuring the integrity of the research process* (Vol. 1). Washington, DC: National Academy Press.

National Academy of Sciences. (1993). *Responsible science: Ensuring the integrity of the research process* (Vol. 2). Washington, DC: National Academy Press.

Nelkin, D. (1983). Whistle blowing and social responsibility in science. *Research ethics.* New York: Alan R. Liss, Inc.

Penslar, R. L. (Ed.). (1995). *Research Ethics. Cases & materials.* Indianapolis: Indiana University Press, 3-12.

Petersdorf, R. G. (1989). A matter of integrity. *Acad Med*, 64, 119-123.

Petersdorf, R. G. (1986). The pathogenesis of fraud in medical science. *Ann Int Med*, 104, 252-254.

Schachman, H. K. (1993). What is misconduct in science? *Science*, 261, 148-149.

Shore, E. G. (1993). Sanctions and remediation for research misconduct: Differential diagnosis, treatment, and prevention. *Acad Med*, 68(Suppl.), S44-S48.

Soskolne, C. L. (Ed.). (1993). Proceedings of the symposium on ethics and law in environmental epidemiology. *J Exp Anal Environ Epidemiol*, 3(Suppl. 1).

Soskolne, C. L. & Macfarlane, D. K. (1996). Scientific misconduct in epidemiologic research. In S. S. Coughlin & T. L. Beauchamp (Eds.). *Ethics and epidemiology* (pp. 274-289). New York: Oxford University Press.

Stewart, W. & Feder, N. (1987). The integrity of the scientific literature. *Nature*, 325, 207-214.

Teich, A. H. & Frankel, M. S. (1992 March). *Good science and responsible scientists: Meeting the challenge of fraud and misconduct in science.* Washington, DC: American Association for the Advancement of Science, American Bar Association, and National Conference of Lawyers and Scientists.

U.S. Department of Health and Human Services. Public Health Service. (1989). Responsibilities of awardee and applicant institutions for dealing with and reporting possible misconduct in science. *Federal Register*, 54, 32446-32451.

Woolf, P. K. (1986). Pressure to publish and fraud in science. *Ann Int Med*, 104, 254-256.

Chapter 7

Conflicting Interests and Research Sponsorship

C onflicting interests occur when one's self-interest is at odds with one's obligations to others. Public health professionals have obligations to follow accepted procedures that can be evaluated by others, to reduce disease morbidity and mortality, to tell the truth, to disseminate findings to achieve the widest possible benefits, and to maintain scientific objectivity. When researchers must choose between such professional obligations and personal gain, they have conflicting interests. In epidemiology, for example, conflicting interests can occur when an epidemiologist makes a judgment about the causality of an association while being financed by interests that might impair his or her objectivity or ability to maintain impartiality.

It is necessary to distinguish *actual* conflicting interests from those that are only potential conflicts, as well as from situations in which there is only the appearance of conflicting interests. For example, if an epidemiologist at an academic medical center accepts an honorarium from a pharmaceutical firm, this might appear to represent conflicting interests—or at least possible conflicting interests—but more information would be required to know whether conflicting interests actually exist.

Researchers who are also physicians, nurses, or other health professionals may have other kinds of conflicting interests. For example, physicians who are offered financial incentives to recruit patients for a clinical trial on a *per capita* basis may encounter a conflict between self-interest and duties to patients and society. Health care professionals traditionally owe their greatest allegiance to their patients. Thus, conflicts may arise in a randomized trial if a patient's therapy may be determined by research funding.

57

The existence of conflicting interests does not necessarily mean that anything improper has occurred. For example, researchers employed by companies that have a financial interest in the results of epidemiologic studies often conduct responsible research. Many reputable scientists work for institutions that receive financial support from parties that have a direct interest in research outcomes.

Concern over possible or actual conflicting interests extends beyond research conducted or funded by private corporations. For example, governments and nongovernmental organizations such as universities and private foundations can also exert undue influence on scientists.

Conflicting interests may be dealt with in a number of ways. It may be possible to eliminate the source of the conflict, such as gifts or side contracts. In other instances, as when a researcher's livelihood depends upon corporate funding, appearances of conflicting interests may be resolved through the consistent performance and reporting of high-quality, objective research. Another approach is to disclose relations that constitute potential conflicting interests. It remains controversial, however, whether disclosures should be required when there is only the appearance of a conflict. Nevertheless, such disclosures do facilitate public scrutiny.

Many corporations, governments, and universities have policies that attempt to address and prevent conflicting interests. Such policies include setting acceptable thresholds for stock ownership in firms for which an employee conducts research. Such policies, when carefully thought out, promulgated, and practiced throughout the institution, can do much to eliminate conflicting interests before they arise.

A number of ethical challenges relating to conflicting interests and research sponsorship are illustrated by the case studies provided in this chapter.

Case 7a: Concern Over Microwave Exposure at the U.S. Embassy in Moscow

Researchers at a major university received a contract from the U.S. Department of State to investigate the possibility of higher than normal cancer risks among workers at the U.S. Embassy in Moscow. There had been concern over exposure from an external source that projected microwave radiation into both the offices and the residential areas of the embassy. This source of radiation first had been recognized in the early 1960s. Between 1966 and 1969, a high mutation rate had been noted in white blood cells obtained from a sample of exposed workers. Later, between 1973 and 1976, significant changes in the blood counts of Moscow employees were documented through comparisons with State Department employees in the United States. The embassy workers were not informed of this exposure until 1976, nor did they receive information about their test results. The exposure was not under the control of the State Department and the intent of those transmitting the radiation was not well understood. The possible adverse health effects also were poorly understood. Disclosing such information could have made the post even less attractive during the Cold War era.

The university researchers completed a large, well-publicized study of the Moscow workers in 1978. The study included State Department employees at other Eastern European embassies as controls, despite evidence that the other embassies also were irradiated. Even so, cancer increases were found in some groups of Moscow employees, and multiple cancers were far more frequent than expected. On the basis of U.S. exposure guidelines at the time of the exposure (but not those of the U.S.S.R.), researchers had not expected significant adverse health effects from the estimated level of microwave radiation exposure.

Descriptive words that might have drawn attention to concern on the part of the investigative team (e.g., "disturbing") were removed from the study report at the request of the contracting officer. Because of the nature of the exposures and their relative recency, the investigative team had recommended that the study population should be contacted at intervals of 2 to 3 years over the next several years, to ascertain if any additional adverse health effects would appear. There was no indication that this recommendation was adopted, which raised concerns over the possibility of a State Department cover-up. After workmen's compensation claims were filed by individual employees, information previously deemed secret or confidential was eventually made available under the Freedom of Information Act.

Questions for Discussion

1.   What are the obligations of the researchers to the workers at the U.S. Embassy in Moscow and to their families? What are the obligations of the researchers to the funding agency? How could the researchers have avoided or resolved these conflicting interests?

2   What ethical concerns are raised by the study design, including the use of controls who also were known to have been exposed?

3.   What additional ethical issues are raised by this study?

Reference

Goldsmith, J. R. (1996). Balancing the interests of patients, science and employees: Case study of RF (microwave) exposures of US embassy staff in Eastern European posts. *Science of the Total Environment*, 184, 83-89.

Case 7b: Cardiovascular Research Sponsored by the Tobacco Industry

A study of the determinants of cardiovascular disease was undertaken by university-based researchers in collaboration with local health departments. Initial funding for the main study was received from the World Health Organization (WHO). The tobacco industry subsequently funded tobacco-related research projects within the overall study.

The researchers soon found themselves faced with demands from tobacco industry sponsors that conflicted with their scientific judgment. The principal investigator, however, refused to yield to any pressure that would have compromised scientific objectivity.

Questions for Discussion

1.   Should the investigators have accepted financial support from the tobacco industry for their cardiovascular research study? What are their obligations to the sponsors in this situation?

2.   Should the institution at which the researchers conducted the research have placed limits on potential sources of support for health-related research?

3.   What safeguards would have been helpful at the time the investigators agreed to accept support from the tobacco industry?

Case 7c: Divulging Research Funding Sources

A number of leading biomedical journals have adopted policies that require authors to divulge their funding sources to editors. Some journals publish this information in conjunction with the publication of scientific reports. The intent behind such policies is to reveal to readers actual or potential conflicting interests. According to one account of why such disclosure is needed, "it is useful for the reader to know who supported a study, when deciding how much credence to give to its conclusions (Sacks et al., 1987, p. 452). Many public health studies are funded by sources that have an interest in the outcome of the studies.

A sharply contrasting viewpoint is that such editorial policies unfairly prejudge such reports by suggesting that the investigators are less than trustworthy. Rothman (1991) has argued that "to prejudge the veracity of scientific work based on investigator characteristics is simply a mistake," and that "to detract from another's findings by appealing to the hidden prejudices that one suspects lurks in his or her mind serves only to defeat open criticism of the science itself. Thus, the ironic result of focusing attention away from the science and toward a perceived conflict of interest is to stifle the objectivity that is desired." (p. 27S)

Questions for Discussion

1.   What role should editors of scientific journals play in identifying conflicting interests of contributors or the appearance of conflicting interests?

2.   What are some of the reasons for worrying about the appearance of conflicting interests?

3.   Do sponsorship disclosure policies unfairly damage the reputations of investigators?

4.   Does the absence of such disclosure jeopardize the validity
or usefulness of the research for health policy-making or secondary analyses such as meta-analysis?

References

Rothman, K. J. (1991). The ethics of research sponsorship. *J Clin Epidemiol*, 44(Suppl. I), 25S-28S.

Sacks, H. S., Berrier, J., Reitman, D., et al. (1987). Meta-analyses of randomized controlled trials. *N Engl J Med*, 316, 450-455.

Case 7d: Conflicting Interests in an Environmental Impact Assessment

In a project jointly sponsored by the African Development
Bank and a local government, a proposed large-scale irrigation
and drainage project was deferred pending the completion of an
environmental impact assessment. An environmental epidemiologist and an outside consulting firm were employed to carry
out the environmental impact assessment. They were to report
their findings to the regional planning office, where the final
decision about whether or not to go ahead with the project was
to be made. At that time, such assessments were a recent innova-
tion in the country and were considered by many to be an
obstacle to development.

In the course of preparing the environmental impact assessment, the research team began to undertake studies assigned
by the regional planning office. It soon became clear to the
epidemiologist that the research team was being encouraged to
produce an assessment favoring the building of the project. The
consulting firm and the companies to which they subcontracted
work undertook the studies in a hurry and seemed unenthusias-
tic about discussing their progress, even unwilling to do so. They
seemed to overlook findings that might have led to a negative
assessment of the project.

When the epidemiologist complained to the regional planning office, he was reassured that it was monitoring all research
projects and that nothing inappropriate was occurring. The office
also emphasized the considerable benefits to the region of having

a water resource project funded by the African Development Bank. The project would bring hundreds of jobs, as well as benefits from the provision of materials for the project and the need to feed and house workers. The regional planning office also cited the regional droughts that had often led to crop failure and famine. Planning officials made it clear to the epidemiologist that they were very hopeful that the environmental impact assessment would come back in favor of the project and that he might expect future work on such projects if everything went smoothly on this initial assessment.

Despite these conflicting interests, the epidemiologist completed his research assignments to the best of his ability, while maintaining his scientific objectivity. He found some evidence of small potential health risks and suggested minor changes to the project to minimize them. The research of the consulting firm also indicated that some minor changes were in order, and all of these recommendations were incorporated into the final environmental impact assessment report. The project continued on schedule as originally planned.

Questions for Discussion

1.   Should stakeholders in a development project—regional planning office—supervise the studies required for an environmental impact assessment?

2.   What responsibility did the African Development Bank, as the primary funding agency, have to ensure the overall integrity of the research leading up to the environmental impact assessment?

3.   To officials in a relatively poor country, public health risks associated with a development project may seem greatly outweighed by the pressing need for development. Whose standards should be applied in such situations—those of the underdeveloped country or those of the international funding agency?

Case 7e: Concern over Peer Review of Government-Sponsored Research

A researcher who had received funding through a government contract submitted study findings to government sponsors for review before submitting the report for publication. This was in compliance with the researcher's contractual agreement with the funding agency. On the basis of what the investigator considered to be a questionable interpretation of the data, the sponsors then suppressed publication of the study results. The researcher was not provided with any opportunity to respond to the critique. Subsequently, the investigator used the study findings to support a research grant application that was rejected. The reasons given for the rejection were vague, and no suggestions were offered to improve the application.

Questions for Discussion

1.   What are the obligations of peer reviewers and funding agencies to researchers, and vice versa?
2.   Do the government sponsors have actual conflicting interests in this situation?

Case 7f: Conflicting Interests in a Study of Occupational Lung Disease

A researcher was conducting a government-funded study of lung disease in a group of industrial workers. The investigator was asked by government officials to present the results of the study to the workers, including the increased risk of lung disease from occupational exposure to dusts. The company agreed to the presentation, but asked the investigator to emphasize the increased risk of lung disease from cigarette smoking and to downplay the role of occupational exposures. The company wished to avoid difficulties with the workers, including the possibility of having to pay financial compensation to affected workers. The researcher hoped that the company would fund a follow-up study as further governmental support was unlikely. The investigator was reluctant to jeopardize future research funding by not respecting the company's request.

Questions for Discussion

1.   What are the professional obligations of the researcher in a situation such as this?

2.   Do the workers have a right to be fully informed about the results of the occupational study, including their risks of disease?

Suggestions for Further Reading

American Council on Education. (1986). Higher education and research entrepreneurship: Conflicts among interests. Washington, DC.

Angell, M. & Kassirer, J. P. (1996). Editorials and conflicts of interest. *New Engl J Med*, 335, 1055-1056.

Anderson, R. E. (1990). The advantages and risks of entrepreneurship. *Academe*, 6, 9-14.

Guidelines for dealing with faculty conflicts of commitment and conflicts of interest in research. (1990). Washington, DC: Association of American Medical Colleges.

Bond, G. G. (1991). Ethical issues relating to the conduct and interpretation of epidemiologic research in private industry. *J Clin Epidemiol*, 44(Suppl. I), 29S-34S.

Bourke, J. & Weissman, R. (1990). Academics at risk: The temptations of profit. *Academe*, 76, 15-21.

Charrow, R. P. (1989). Weighing conflict solutions to conflict of interest. *J NIH Research*, 1, 138-139.

Friedman, P. J. (1991). Controlling conflict of interests. *Issues in Science and Technology*, 8, 30-32.

Kassirer, J. P. & Angell, M. (1993). Financial conflicts of interest in biomedical research. *New Engl J Med*, 329, 570-571.

Korenman, S. G. (1993). Conflicts of interest and commercialization of research. *Acad Med*, 68(Suppl.), S18-S22.

Korenman, S. G. & Shipp, A. C. (1994). Teaching the responsible conduct of research through a case study approach. A handbook for instructors. Washington, DC: Association of American Medical Colleges.

Kreiser, B. R. (1990). On preventing conflicts of interest in government sponsored research at universities. In *AAUP policy documents and reports* (7th ed.). Washington, DC: American Association of University Professors.

Macrina, F. L. (1995). *Scientific integrity. An introductory text with cases.* Washington, DC: American Society for Microbiology.

Marshall, E. (1990). When commerce and academe collide. *Science,* 248, 152-156.

Porter, R. J. & Malone, T. E. (1992). *Biomedical research: Collaboration and conflict of interest.* Baltimore, MD: The Johns Hopkins University Press.

Relman, A. S. (1984). Dealing with conflicts of interest. *N Engl J Med,* 310, 1182-1183.

Soskolne, C. L. (1985). Epidemiological research, interest groups and the review process. *J Public Health Policy,* 7, 173-184.

Soskolne, C. L. (1989). Epidemiology: Questions of science, ethics, morality, and law. *Am J Epidemiol,* 129, 1-18.

Stolley, P. D. (1991). Ethical issues involving conflicts of interest for epidemiologic investigators. A report of the Committee on Ethical Guidelines of the Society for Epidemiologic Research. *J Clin Epidemiol,* 44(Suppl. I), 23S-24S.

Thompson, D. C. (1993). Understanding financial conflicts of interest. *N Engl J Med,* 329, 573-576.

Chapter 8

Intellectual Property and Data Sharing

The history of science (including that of applied sciences such as public health disciplines) is rich with examples of sacrifice, heroism, and generosity, but also with episodes of greed, selfishness, and disputes over attribution, recognition, and compensation. Competition and pride among scientists have both spurred the growth of knowledge and, on occasion, reflected poorly on investigators and their institutions. Disputes over intellectual property rights have often been at the heart of such controversies.

The very idea of intellectual property strikes some as oxymoronic—how can notions of property be applied to ideas? The theft or appropriation of intellectual property does not usually deprive the "owner" or discoverer of the use of a novel idea. Instead, what is lost is *control* over the idea. There are a number of reasons why someone would want to control communication about an idea. These often boil down to questions of recognition (e.g., who discovered an idea first) and remuneration, if not outright fame and fortune. Loss of control over ideas can deprive the discoverer or creator of an idea of appropriate compensation or just rewards for his or her insight.

Nevertheless, communities of scientists—and society in general—are enriched by the practice of scientific publishing and the dissemination of research findings. Thus, the rights of those who come up with a new idea or discovery first must be balanced against the need to avoid unduly restricting or controlling others' use of the idea.

In public health and other fields, the practice of sharing scientific data and health information can give rise to ethical conflicts. Researchers may be motivated to refrain from sharing data in order to protect financial interests, to enhance their standing in the field, or, worse yet, to impede the work of others. Or they may fear potential harms or risks to research participants. Many data sets in epidemiology and public health, for example, contain confidential information that must be carefully protected. Nevertheless, the failure to share data can lead to the wasting of scarce resources or prevent worthwhile forms of research.

Disputes over intellectual property and data sharing often are caused or worsened by the failure to communicate effectively. Research institutions, individual researchers, and funding agencies need to develop written policies about intellectual property rights and the sharing of data so that misunderstandings and conflicts can be reduced or avoided.

A number of ethical issues related to intellectual property disputes are highlighted in the cases presented in this chapter.

Case 8a: Conflicts between Colleagues at a University

A published research project attracted the interest of a newly appointed faculty member of a large department of epidemiology. The new faculty member had worked in a related area of research and was interested in acquiring the raw data from the faculty member who had completed the study with support from industry. The faculty member was provided with copies of the data set and project coding manual.

Within a month, it came to the attention of the faculty member who had provided the data that her new colleague had submitted a grant application to a public funding agency in which the data set had been committed to the establishment of a comparative database. This was to be made possible by virtue of access to the full data set, permitting various subgroupings of the data. The individual who had provided the data set had not been invited to participate in the development of the grant application.

Questions for Discussion

1.   Should the faculty member who had developed the initial data set have made it available to her newly appointed colleague

in the first place? Should there have been explicit understandings between them about how the data set would be handled? What points ought to have been communicated? Should these points have been in writing, or is a verbal understanding adequate in a situation like this?

2. Before handing over copies of the data to her new colleague, should the faculty member have first secured permission from the industrial sponsors of her study?

3. What are the rights and responsibilities of faculty members regarding the storing and sharing of data from industry-sponsored research (or research funded by a public agency) that is undertaken at an academic institution?

Case 8b: Concern over Plagiarism by a Department Chair

A junior faculty member at a university became concerned that he was being asked to borrow material improperly from a paper reviewed by the chairperson of his department as part of the peer review process. The chair had reviewed the paper as an anonymous referee. The junior faculty member had heard the paper presented orally at a scientific conference a few months earlier. He believed that the chair was borrowing information from the paper without permission to improve her chances of securing funding for a research grant application that was about to be submitted to a funding agency. The junior faculty member was listed as a co-investigator on the draft grant application.

The information that the chair wished to use in the preparation of the grant application included findings from the paper under review as well as a portion of its literature review and methodology. The chair had instructed the junior faculty member to integrate this material into the grant application as it was developed.

Questions for Discussion

1. Should the junior faculty member comply with the chair's request? Whose interests does the junior faculty member have an obligation to protect?

2.   Should the junior faculty member confront the chair with his concerns over plagiarism or should he first report the chair's actions to a third party?

3.   What are the rights and obligations of the department chair in a situation such as this?

Case 8c: Court Case Involving Plagiarism of an Epidemiologic Study Questionnaire

In what is apparently the world's first legal determination that a scientist was guilty of plagiarism, courts ruled that an epidemiologist violated a copyright and made inappropriate use of confidential information.

The 7-year court battle focused on the development of questionnaires designed to study the incidence of lung cancer in nonsmoking women. Over a nearly 2-year period, two researchers drafted 14 versions of a questionnaire, the final version of which contained 69 core questions and many secondary questions. A third researcher, working on the same research question but under a separate grant, later produced four drafts of another questionnaire. The first two investigators alleged that the third appropriated parts of their questionnaire. The third admitted having a copy of their questionnaire, but initially denied using any part of it as his own, and in any event said that the two others had given him the copy. He later admitted to some use of the first questionnaire.

Testimony at trial addressed the similarities and differences between the questionnaires and included a linguist as an expert witness. One authority insisted that epidemiologists often share information about questionnaires, and that questionnaires were not the sorts of things that should be subjected to copyright protection.

As a complicating factor, one of the first two investigators has alleged that she was penalized as a whistleblower: She remained a lecturer for 13 years, whereas her rival was promoted during the trial.

Questions for Discussion

1.   Should scientific instruments such as questionnaires be copyrighted or otherwise protected as intellectual property?

2.   To what extent do scientists have an obligation to share information such as questionnaires with colleagues? If an investigator declines to share such information, is it permissible to go ahead and use it anyway?

3.   What kind of professional norms or institutional policies might be helpful for preventing conflicts such as the one outlined in this case?

Reference

Swinbanks, D. (1993). Survey battle leads to plagiarism verdict. *Nature, 366,* 715.

Suggestions for Further Reading

Barrett, M. (1991). *Intellectual Property.* Larchmount, NY: Emanuel Law Outlines.

Chalmers, I. (1990). Underreporting research is scientific misconduct. *JAMA, 263,* 1405-1408.

Estabrooks, C. A. & Romyn, D. M. (1995). Data sharing in nursing research: Advantages and challenges. *Can J Nurs Res, 27,* 77-88.

Fayerweather, W. E., Tirey, S. L., Baldwin, J. K. & Hoover, B. K. (1991). Issues in data sharing and access: An industry perspective. *J Occup Med, 33,*1253-1256.

Fienberg, S. E. (1994). Sharing statistical data in the biomedical and health sciences: ethical, institutional, legal, and professional dimensions. *Ann Rev Public Health, 15,* 1-18.

Foltz, R. & Penn, T. (1990). *Protecting scientific ideas and inventions.* Boca Raton, FL: CRC Press.

Goldman, A. H. (1987). Ethical issues in proprietary restrictions on research results. *Sci Tech Human Values, 1,* 22-30.

Goodman, K. (1993). Intellectual property and control. *Acad Med, 68,* S88-91.

Hogue, C. J. R. (1991). Ethical issues in sharing epidemiologic data. *J Clin Epidemiol, 44*(Suppl. I), 103S-107S.

Korenman, S. G. & Shipp, A. C. (1994). *Teaching the responsible conduct of research through a case study approach. A handbook for instructors.* Washington, DC: Association of American Medical Colleges.

Macrina, F. L. (1995). *Scientific Integrity. An introductory text with cases.* Washington, DC: American Society for Microbiology.

Marshall, E. (1990). Data sharing: A declining ethic? *Science,* 248, 952-957.

Miller, A. & Davis R. (1990). *Intellectual property—patents, trademarks, and copyright in a nutshell* (2nd ed.). St. Paul, MN: West Publishing Co.

Fineberg, S. E., Martin, M. E. & Straf, M. L. (Eds.). (1985). *Sharing research data.* Washington, DC: National Academy Press.

Yolles, B. J., Connors, J. C. & Grufferman, S. (1986). Obtaining access to data from government-sponsored medical research. *N Engl J Med,* 315, 1669-1672.

Chapter 9

Publication and Interpretation of Research Findings

One way to reflect on scientific progress in public health and other fields is to look for the accumulation of truths, identification of solutions to problems, or the development of methods for learning about the world. Reports of these changes are sometimes conceived of as residing in a *corpus,* a body of belief. A corpus serves several vital functions: It represents the status of a science at a given point; it allows what is known—or believed—to be shared among scientists and transmitted to students and society; and it serves as a platform from which to launch new investigations. A scientific corpus also helps individuals and teams to be acknowledged for their work. The corpus undergoes constant change. As new studies and observations are completed, reports about them add to the corpus or displace earlier reports. A corpus may contain conflicting, even contradictory reports, although not indefinitely.

Contributions to the scientific literature also serve a variety of social and economic functions. Jobs, promotions (including academic tenure), financial support, and other benefits often are awarded because these contributions are numerous, of high quality, or of great importance.

This discussion underscores the important role that publication and authorship play in scientific progress. It also illuminates why disputes and controversies about publication and authorship are among the most common in academic, corporate, government, and other research. The stakes can be relatively high.

It is important to make students and practicing public health professionals aware of clear cases of misconduct related to publication and authorship, including those related to plagiarism, fabrication, and falsification of data. It also is crucial for them to be aware that not all cases are clear-cut, and that reasonable people might disagree about criteria for assigning and ordering authorship, avoiding redundant publication, and the like. When we err about publication and authorship, we sully or pollute the scientific corpus. This impedes the research enterprise and harms both society and individual researchers.

A corpus can also be corrupted by omissions. The well-known problem of publication bias results when scientists and editors do not accord proper weight to studies that fail to show positive results. This misleads researchers and policy makers who need to obtain a complete and accurate picture of results in a given area. Publication bias is particularly harmful ·to meta-analyses, the conduct of which increases the obligations of researchers to produce timely, accurate, and complete reports of their work.

Difficult ethical tensions also can arise between students and their mentors. Students often are unclear about what efforts are sufficient to warrant co-authorship. Mentors are sometimes accused of taking advantage of students.

Ethical conflicts about publication can be reduced by making criteria and guidelines for publication readily available. The establishment of ground rules for publication and authorship should come at the start of a research project, not after a conflict or misunderstanding has emerged. A number of such conflicts are described in the case studies that follow.

Case 9a: Authorship Credit

(This case study, which comes from course materials developed by Ronald Prineas and Kenneth Goodman, is included here in revised form with the permission of the authors.)

A newly appointed assistant professor proposed a hypothesis to be tested with ecological data to the chair of her department and suggested that they collaborate on collection of data and reporting of the analysis. Letters written by the chair (at the behest of the assistant professor), greatly expedited data collection from government agencies and private industry because of the chair's authority and name recognition.

In the course of time, data analysis and figures were prepared for a report. The analyses, the figures, and a table were submitted to the chair for comment along with an indication that the first paper draft would follow. The chair had no suggestion for different or additional analyses.

Two months passed without a draft being readied and without discussion of the paper between the assistant professor and chair. At the end of this period the assistant professor took a two-week vacation. When she returned, the chair presented her with a draft of the paper with the chair listed as first author and the assistant professor listed second. The assistant professor felt cheated of first authorship but said nothing. The assistant professor made format and editorial changes to the paper and added further reference material and explication to the discussion section of the paper. The paper was submitted, accepted, and published.

Questions for Discussion

1.   Was the conduct of either the chair or the assistant professor unethical?
2.   What course of action would you have taken if you were the assistant professor?
3.   What would your reply have been if you were the chair and the assistant professor had stated (before submission of the article) that she should be first author because she had conceived the project, collected much of the data, and carried out the analyses?

Case 9b: Potential Conflict over Order of Authorship

A potential conflict arose over a report stemming from an epidemiological study of childhood cancer and parental exposure to carcinogens. The study was conducted by a nontenured assistant professor of epidemiology at a university hospital and a doctoral candidate under his supervision. The assistant professor had designed the study, supervised the graduate student, and made revisions to the manuscript. The graduate student had undertaken the management and coordination of the project, and had done the majority of the writing of the manuscript. The assistant professor believed that the graduate student should have the distinction of being first author, both because she had done most of the work and because it would be advantageous for her career.

Tension arose when the head of the department insisted that the assistant professor's name be placed first because the assistant professor had designed the study. The department head also contended that it would be more beneficial to the department and the university hospital to have the results of this important study published under the assistant professor's name rather than that of an unknown graduate student. The assistant professor, who was under consideration for tenure, believed that his position in the department would be more secure if he were to publish this paper as first author. The assistant professor then discussed the matter with the graduate student, and they agreed that, given the departmental situation, it was in everyone's best interest to place the assistant professor's name first. They agreed that in the future they would reach a decision about the order of authorship before the work began, based upon who would play the most important role in carrying out the research.

Questions for Discussion

1.   What criteria should be used to determine the order of authorship in health research?
2.   Did the assistant professor's role in designing the study and supervising the graduate student justify placing his name first on the manuscript?
3.   In this case, the issue was resolved without substantial conflict, and the relationship between the graduate student and the professor was undamaged. If a conflict had occurred, how might it have been resolved in an equitable fashion?

Case 9c: Claims to Honorary Coauthorship by a Department Head

A promising young researcher was hired as an associate professor at a department of public health. Within her first two years, she produced some excellent papers based upon research she conducted with a research associate. The head of the department was impressed by the quality of the research and attempted to claim coauthorship on the manuscripts based on his academic rank and seniority. He even implied that if his name did not appear on the papers, the associate professor would have no chance of advancement within the department as long as he had any say in the matter. The associate professor approached the associate dean of the faculty to bring the matter to his attention. After a meeting with the associate dean in which the department head was confronted with the issue, the department head withdrew his "request" for coauthorship.

Questions for Discussion

1.   Are there any circumstances in which "honorary coauthorship" should be extended to a department head who has not made a contribution to a paper? Did the administrative role of the department head justify placing his name on the manuscript?
2.   What criteria should be used to determine coauthorship in health research?
3.   Did the researcher act properly in approaching the associate dean about the department head's claims to authorship?

Case 9d: Pressure To Go Beyond the Limits of the Data

Urban mortality studies conducted by epidemiologists, demographers, and other researchers often contribute to the formulation of social and health policy. Urban planners draw upon the findings of such studies to enhance the quality of life for urban residents. Although mortality data from epidemiologic studies often form the basis for rational policymaking, other factors influence the formulation of public policy. These include economic factors, religious values, and political pressures.

A recent example occurred when a group of epidemiologists undertook comparative mortality studies in two urban populations. The research was sponsored by an environmental policy department. The members of the research team included the epidemiologists, government officials, members of municipal health departments, and statisticians. Urban planners in the sponsoring groups also played a role.

In the course of these multidisciplinary studies, a conflict arose between the health researchers and the urban planners. From the perspective of the researchers, the urban planners were seeking simplistic solutions to complex interactions among various health determinants. The researchers felt pressured to interpret their data beyond what they believed the scientific method and inference would allow. In their view, the policy makers seemed to be responding more to political expediency than to sound science. The collaborators also found it difficult to understand the jargon of each others' discipline.

Questions for Discussion

1.   How should researchers respond when they feel pressured to overinterpret their results or to oversimplify scientific relationships? To what extent do epidemiologists and other researchers have an ethical obligation to communicate their work in ways that are understandable to others?

2.   What obligations do epidemiologists have to stakeholders outside the profession such as public planners, policy makers, and politicians?

Case 9e: Questionable Analysis of the Data by a Principal Investigator

A study was conducted to examine the prevalence of elevated lead levels in children living in homes and schools with lead-containing paints or plastic blinds covered with lead dust. The study was jointly conducted by government agencies and a private consulting group. The principal investigator was eager to show a correlation between these two exposures and elevated lead levels in the children tested. When appropriate data analysis methods were applied, the researchers were unable to show any correlation. The principal investigator then changed the method of data analysis in order to obtain the desired results. Although one of the junior investigators objected to the practices of the principal investigator, the revised study results were released anyway. The junior investigator informed government officials of the inappropriate method of data analysis, but the officials were unwilling to take any vigorous action that might have jeopardized the reputation of their agency. They did, however, quietly voice their concerns to the principal investigator, who soon left the project.

Questions for Discussion
1.   Did the junior investigator behave properly by "blowing the whistle" on the principal investigator?
2.   What mechanisms are in place for whistleblowers to report allegations of improper research practices and for institutions or agency officials to respond to such allegations?
3.   Did the officials at the government agency behave properly when they failed to respond vigorously to the information provided by the junior investigator?

Case 9f: Omission of Out-of-Range Values in an Environmental Health Study

A group of industrial workers was tested for levels of a specific biomarker that would indicate their exposure levels to dioxins. The well-designed study was funded and conducted jointly by a government in Europe and by industry. The principal investigator instructed one of the researchers to omit certain high values, pointing out that they "must be errors." The researcher refused to change any of the values, however. He believed that the principal investigator was allowing industry representatives, who had strong feelings about the outcome of the study, to influence his perception and to compromise his objectivity.

Questions for Discussion

1.   Was the principal investigator tampering with the data by instructing that the high values be omitted, or was he exercising sound scientific judgment?
2.   What actions should the researcher take in this situation to meet his professional responsibilities?

Suggestions for Further Reading

Angell, M. (1986). Publish or perish: A proposal. *Ann Int Med*, 104, 261-262.

Altman, D. G. (1980). Statistics and ethics in medical research: Misuse of statistics is unethical. *Br Med J*, 281, 1182-1184.

Caelleigh, A. S. (1991). Credit and responsibility in authorship [Editorial]. *Academic Medicine*, 66, 676-677.

Chalmers, I. (1990). Underreporting research is scientific misconduct. *JAMA*, 263, 1405-1408.

Council of Biology Editors Editorial Policy Committee. (1990). *Ethics and policy in scientific publications*. Bethesda, MD: Council of Biology Editors.

Dickersin, K. & Min, Y. I. (1993). Publication bias: The problem that won't go away. In K. W. Wachter & F. Mosteller (Eds.), *Doing more good than harm: The evaluation of health care interventions* (pp. 135-146). New York: New York Academy of Sciences.

Fye, W. B. (1990). Medical authorship: traditions, trends, and tribulations. *Ann Int Med*, 113, 317-325.

Glass, R. M. (1992). New information for authors and readers: Group authorship, acknowledgements, and rejected manuscripts [Editorial]. *JAMA*, 268, 99.

Huth, E. J. (1986). Abuses and uses of authorship. *Ann Int Med*, 104, 266-267.

Huth, E. J. (1986). Guidelines on authorship of medical papers. *Ann Int Med*, 104, 269-274.

Korenman, S. G. & Shipp, A. C. (1994). *Teaching the responsible conduct of research through a case study approach. A handbook for instructors*. Washington, DC: Association of American Medical Colleges.

Macrina, F. L. (1995). *Scientific integrity. An introductory text with cases.* Washington, DC: American Society for Microbiology.

National Academy of Sciences. (1993). *Responsible science: Vol. II. Ensuring the integrity of the research process.* Washington, DC: National Academy Press.

Penslar, R. L. (Ed.). (1995). *Research ethics. Cases & materials.* Indianapolis: Indiana University Press.

Relman, A. S. (1990). Publishing biomedical research: Roles and responsibilities. *Hastings Center Rep, 20,* 23-27.

Riesenberg, D. & Lundberg, G. D. (1990). The order of authorship: Who's on first? [Editorial]. *JAMA, 264,* 1857.

Shapiro, S. (1985). The decision to publish. Ethical dilemmas. *J Chron Dis, 38,* 365-372.

Soskolne, C. L. (Ed.). (1993). Ethics and law in environmental epidemiology. *J Exp Anal Environ Epidemiol, 3*(Suppl. 1), 243-320.

Szklo, M. (1991). Issues in publication and interpretation of research findings. *J Clin Epidemiol, 44,* 109S-113S.

Chapter 10

Communication Responsibilities of Public Health Professionals

O ne of the most challenging areas of public health ethics is determining the extent to which scientists and policy makers have an obligation to disclose risks and other scientific data. From causes of cancer to environmental exposures to Creutzfeldt-Jakob Disease and bovine spongiform encephalopathy (or "mad cow disease"), the consequences of speaking too late—or too soon—can be very great indeed. These challenges are many times magnified when we interject issues of public policy, intercultural communication, and social advocacy by scientists.

It is not enough to insist that public health professionals must always "tell the truth," especially when the truth is unknown or uncertain. Proof or certainty might not be available until after the damage is done.

The problem here is shaped in part by the fact that public health professionals rarely communicate directly with the people affected by their work. Public health and epidemiologic findings are customarily communicated broadly through various news media, which take their cues from direct contact with investigators, from presentations at scientific meetings, from the peer-reviewed scientific literature, and from other sources.

A further challenge is that many people are overwhelmed by what they perceive to be a vast and potentially contradictory body of research on various potential and actual health hazards. It is not clear in such a context that more information will produce greater understanding.

Nevertheless, the potential benefits of disclosing health information tend to outweigh those of remaining silent. Fears that one's message will be misunderstood tend to produce a chilling effect that can impede research, diminish trust, and erode support for the scientific enterprise. Public health professionals have an important obligation to use caution and sound judgment in informing people who are affected by public health research. Stakeholder groups include affected communities, professional colleagues, and courts of law.

Case 10a: Expert Testimony on Causality and the Role of Epidemiologists in Court

Occupational epidemiologists determine the relationship between workplace exposures and disease occurrence. Information obtained from such studies is used in addressing issues of workers' compensation and third-party liability through review boards and the judicial system. Occupational epidemiologists and occupational physicians often are asked to testify as expert witnesses when the causes of work-related illnesses are in dispute. Many epidemiologic studies, however, do not produce conclusive evidence about causation.

The uncertainty of etiology and the difficulty of communicating epidemiologic concepts to lay persons can give rise to ethical dilemmas in professional practice. For example, an epidemiologist recently served as an expert witness in a court case concerning a purported excess of cancer mortality in an industrial plant. The plant had a known history of substantial asbestos use without any protection against worker exposure. A team of expert witnesses had been assembled by the lawyers representing the next-of-kin of a former worker who had died of cancer. The team included a coroner, occupational physicians, industrial engineers and chemists, and the epidemiologist.

A retrospective cancer mortality study had been conducted for the cohort of workers exposed to the asbestos. No deaths from pleural mesothelioma were known to have occurred, although the number of such deaths expected was small. The observed-to-expected (O/E) ratio of lung cancer deaths was 1.2, based upon four observed deaths (where an O/E ratio of 1.0 implies "no association"). The O/E ratio for deaths from cancer of the digestive tract (esophagus, stomach, and large intestine combined) was about 2.0 (12 observed deaths compared to 6.1 expected deaths). This apparent twofold increase in deaths attributed to cancer of the digestive tract was statistically of borderline significance. On the basis of these data, the epidemiologist was asked to give an opinion about whether or not exposure to asbestos in this workplace was responsible for the observed cancer deaths.

The epidemiologist was aware that a large body of scientific evidence has implicated asbestos exposure in the etiology of mesothelioma and lung cancer, although other factors may have a role. The weight of the evidence also suggests that asbestos exposure can cause cancer of the digestive tract, although there have been some inconsistencies across studies.

Questions for Discussion

1.   What opinion should the epidemiologist have given about whether exposure to asbestos was responsible for the observed cancer deaths?
2.   How should the epidemiologist have weighed the need to ensure adequate compensation for the deceased workers' next-of-kin against the need to tell the truth and explain the uncertainty of the scientific evidence about causation?
3.   To what extent was the epidemiologist obligated to explain the limitations of epidemiologic studies and the potential weaknesses of causal inference from observational (nonexperimental) data?

Case 10b: Concern over Delay in Releasing Results of a Study of Childhood Cancer

Members of a community became concerned over what they perceived to be a high rate of childhood cancer. In response to their concerns, university-based researchers undertook a study of childhood cancer and residence in proximity to industrial facilities. The study was funded by a governmental agency under a contractual agreement.

The researchers wished to report the findings of the study to members of the community in a timely fashion. However, a conflict arose between the researchers' desire to report the findings soon after completion of the research and the funding agency's request that reporting of the findings be delayed. The public release of the report was postponed. The researchers believed that the delay was the result of conflicting interests within the government agency. Bureaucratic inefficiency also may have played a role. It was only after extensive lobbying by influential researchers that the governmental agency finally agreed to release the findings.

Questions for Discussion

1.   What are the obligations of the researchers to members of the local community and to the funding agency?
2.   Under what circumstances is it permissible or obligatory for researchers to advocate on behalf of members of a community?
3.   Should the investigators have undertaken the research in the absence of a written agreement with the funding agency about how the release of the study's findings would be timed?

Case 10c: Duty to Inform Participants of Research Results in a Study of Dry-Cleaning Workers

A team of environmental and occupational epidemiologists was commissioned by a regional health authority to study the possibility that exposure to perchloroethylene in the dry-cleaning process posed health hazards. The epidemiologists found evidence of early neurological changes in color vision among a small sample of the workers. A number of the workers exposed to low levels of perchloroethylene experienced temporary loss of color vision, but their vision always returned to normal within 15 minutes of leaving work areas. There was no evidence that the effect was permanent.

The epidemiologists were not surprised by their findings since perchloroethylene is known to affect the central nervous system and to cause eye irritation. They postulated that the temporary loss of color vision was caused by occasional exposure to relatively high doses of perchloroethylene mist, which could be avoided by paying closer attention to existing safety procedures. The research team submitted its results to the companies involved, but not to the individual workers. The epidemiologists believed there was no need to alarm the workers since the employers were doing all they could to ensure that high-dose exposures did not recur. Since the sample size was not large enough for them to draw conclusions with great certainty or precision, the researchers believed that it would be irresponsible for them to disseminate preliminary results widely and risk damaging the companies involved.

Eight weeks later, some of the workers were hospitalized, complaining of complete loss of color vision, blurred vision, and headaches. The attending physicians believed the visual damage to be permanent. What the research team had assumed to be a temporary effect turned out to have long-term adverse consequences for some of the workers.

Questions for Discussion

1.   Should the researchers have warned the dry-cleaning workers of the possibility that they would be harmed by exposure to perchloroethylene?

2.   What factors should be considered in deciding whether or not to inform study participants of a potential risk?

Case 10d: Heavy-Metal Contamination of Produce in a Community

A study was undertaken to examine the amount of heavy metals in regularly consumed foods in a community. The university-based research team was supported by government funding. The investigators found marginally high levels of heavy metals in a variety of fresh produce that was grown by a local farming cooperative. Although the investigators wanted to release the results of the study publicly, the government sponsors were concerned about the potential economic impact on the community. The investigators postponed the release of the study findings to the public so that the farming cooperative could be informed about the problem and given the opportunity to reduce the amount of heavy metals in the soil (and consequently in the produce). This delay in informing the public about the study results was also intended to prevent public panic and protect the economic interests of the community.

Questions for Discussion

1.   What are the obligations of the investigators to the community affected by the heavy-metal contamination? To the government sponsors? To the farming cooperative? How should the investigators have met these obligations?

2.   Did the researchers compromise their obligation to communicate the results of their study in a timely fashion by postponing the release of the study results to the affected community?

3.   Who should the investigators have informed first about the results of the study: the government sponsors, the farming cooperative, the affected community, or the scientific community? Should the investigators have submitted their report to rigorous scientific peer review before informing the community about the results of the study?

Case 10e: Disclosure of Information about Asbestos Health Risks to the Public

Environmental exposure to asbestos has become an important public health concern in many countries. Much of the epidemiologic evidence concerning the health risks of asbestos stems from studies of occupationally exposed workers and their families. Because these workers were exposed to relatively high levels of asbestos, there has been some uncertainty about the health risks posed by ambient levels of asbestos in specific nonoccupational environments. In some countries, asbestos has been removed from schools and other public buildings to minimize risks to children and others.

Highlighting such concerns, a public school recently sponsored a program to develop public health messages about the potential dangers of asbestos exposure and the need for asbestos clean-up and removal. The program was jointly funded by the national health system and a nonprofit private organization. The team of experts charged with developing the health messages included an occupational health physician, an epidemiologist, psychologists, health educators, teachers, and students from a local technical school.

Difficulties soon arose in developing the asbestos risk information messages. These related to scientific uncertainty about the potential risks and benefits of asbestos removal and the need to communicate clear, definitive information to the public. There were conflicting expert opinions about how to remedy the problem of existing asbestos in public buildings. The team of public health professionals was faced with the problem of how best to communicate health risks in the presence of scientific uncertainty.

Questions for Discussion

1.   What information, if any, should be conveyed to the public about potential health risks when there is scientific uncertainty about the risks or about how best to minimize those risks?

2.   Would it be overly paternalistic to withhold information from the public regarding the possible benefits of asbestos removal, given current scientific uncertainty?

Case 10f: Media Accounts of Mad Cow Disease and Consumer Panic in Britain

Driven in part by scientific reports about the incidence of bovine spongiform encephalopathy in British cattle, and partly by popular press reports of "mad cow disease," 1.4 million British households stopped buying beef in late 1995. The British government issued a number of statements intended to reassure people about the safety of the food supply and to point out that no link had been identified between the animal disease and Creutzfeldt-Jakob Disease, a rare neurological disease often fatal in humans.

There are about 11.8 million cattle in the United Kingdom. The rate of bovine spongiform encephalopathy, which was 900 to 1,000 cases per week in 1992, had declined to about 300 cases per week by 1995. Epidemiologists reported that the rate of Creutzfeldt-Jakob Disease in humans, while quite low, had been increasing in Britain. Concern by epidemiologists over this trend was reported in the popular press. The beef industry denied that there was any link between bovine spongiform encephalopathy and accused the media of sensationalism.

Then, in early 1996, investigators in Edinburgh reported 10 human cases of a variant of Creutzfeldt-Jakob Disease and concluded the "most likely" cause was that the 10 individuals ate contaminated beef before a 1989 ban on meat and bone meal in the cattle food supply. There was, in fact, no evidence that these individuals had consumed contaminated beef. Other scientists warned of a vast, deadly epidemic.

What followed was a temporary collapse of the $6.5 billion British beef industry, extraordinary tensions in the European Union (which experienced a 20 to 30 percent drop in beef consumption and a complete ban on British beef and by-products), and evidence of concern as far away as North and South America. This case—variously described as a "crisis," "debacle," and "catastrophe"—was all the more dramatic because of the way the original scientific reports were conveyed by the popular press and handled by the British government.

Questions for Discussion

1.   Some public health reports have economic consequences that can affect the lives of many individuals. How should epidemiologists and public health officials take this into account in communicating information to colleagues, government agencies, and the news media?
2.   Should epidemiologists and public health officials consider the possible impact of their reported studies as conveyed and interpreted by the media?
3.   In evaluating and interpreting health risks, how should public understanding of risk and scientific uncertainty be taken into account?

References

Boffey, P. M. (1996, March 29). Are the mad cows bad cows? *The New York Times*, p. A12.

Darnton, J. (1996, January 1). Fear of mad-cow disease spoils Britain's appetite. *The New York Times*, p. A1.

Darnton, J. (1996, March 28). Europe orders ban on British exports of beef products. *The New York Times,* pp. A1, A8.

Suggestions for Further Reading

Black, B. & Lilienfeld, D. E. (1984). Epidemiologic proof in toxic tort litigation. *Fordham Law Rev,* 52, 732-785.

Cole, P. (1991). The epidemiologist as an expert witness. *J Clin Epidemiol,* 44, 35S-40S.

Cothern, C. A. (Ed.) (1996). *Handbook for environmental risk decision making: Values, perceptions, & ethics.* Boca Raton, FL: CRC Press, pp. 103-113.

Higginson, J. & Chu, F. (1991). Ethical considerations and responsibilities in communicating health risk information. *J Clin Epidemiol,* 44(Suppl. I), 51S-56S.

Jamieson, D. (1996). Scientific uncertainty: How do we know when to communicate research findings to the public? *Science of the Total Environment,* 184, 103-108.

Jonsen, A. R. (1991). Ethical considerations and responsibilities when communicating health risk information. *J Clin Epidemiol,* 44(Suppl. I), 69S-72S.

National Institute for Occupational Safety and Health. (1990). NIOSH pocket guide to chemical hazards. Washington, DC: U.S. Department of Health and Human Services.

Poole, C. & Rothman, K. J. (1990). Epidemiologic science and public health policy (letter). *J Clin Epidemiol,* 43, 1270.

Rothman, K. J. & Poole, C. (1985). Science and policy making [Editorial]. *Am J Public Health,* 75, 340-341.

Sandman, P. M. (1991). Emerging communication responsibilities of epidemiologists. *J Clin Epidemiol,* 44(Suppl. I), 41S-50S.

Schulte, P. A. (1991). Ethical issues in the communication of results. *J Clin Epidemiol,* 44(Suppl. I), 57S-61S.

Schulte, P. A. & Singal, M. (1996). Ethical issues in the interaction with subjects and disclosure of results. In S. S. Coughlin & T. L. Beauchamp (Eds), *Ethics and epidemiology* (pp. 178-196). New York: Oxford University Press.

Soskolne, C. L., Lilienfeld, D. & Black, B. (1996). Epidemiology in legal proceedings in the United States. In M. A. Mehlman & A. Upton, (Eds.), *Advances in modern environmental toxicology.*

Vol. XXII. The identification and control of environmental and occupational diseases: asbestos and cancers (pp. 101-115). Princeton, NJ: Princeton Scientific Publishing Company, Inc.

Spivey, G. H. (1991). Health risk communication—A view from within industry. *J Clin Epidemiol*, 44(Suppl. I), 63S-67S.

Wartenberg, D. (1994). *Epidemiology for journalists*. Los Angeles: Foundation for American Communications.

Weed, D. L. (1994). Science, ethics guidelines, and advocacy in epidemiology. *Ann Epidemiol*, 4, 166-171.

Winsten, J. (1996). Do's and don'ts in dealing with the press. *Epidemiology Monitor*, 17, 10-11, 15.

Yankauer, A. (1984). Science and social policy. *Am J Public Health*, 74, 1148-1149.

Chapter 11

Public Health Practice

In most countries, public health measures that protect against the spread of communicable diseases are addressed by government regulations and legislation. Public health practitioners often have a legal mandate, for example, to inspect food preparation areas in restaurants and, if necessary, to close a restaurant to protect the public. Under certain circumstances, public health officers can even quarantine individuals who put the health of the community at risk.

In carrying out such activities, public health practitioners must balance the need to promote the common welfare against autonomy-based rights of individuals such as freedom of movement or expectations of privacy. In public health laws, however, principles such as beneficence and utility often carry more weight than do principles of autonomy. Water fluoridation programs are another example of a public health intervention in which collective good takes precedence over individual freedom to choose. Likewise, in many towns and municipalities, public water supplies are treated to prevent the transmission of enteric diseases. Other examples of this tendency include legal mandates for the reporting of communicable diseases, disease registries and surveillance systems, vaccination programs for childhood diseases, and contact tracing for the control of sexually transmitted diseases.

Public health laws often cover not only infectious diseases such as AIDS, tuberculosis, and sexually transmitted diseases, but also chronic diseases such as coronary heart disease, diabetes, cancer, birth defects, and even intentional and unintentional injuries. Registries for the surveillance of cancer, for example, are required by law in many parts of the world. To protect confidentiality, data from such registries and surveillance systems must be rigorously protected from unauthorized access.

Public health professionals in whom such powers are vested are usually medical officers trained in preventive medicine, epidemiology, bacteriology, and related fields. They must keep abreast of the most recent scientific information, safeguard the public's health, and provide input to policy makers and legislators who often are influenced by political, economic, and community interests.

Public health education programs such as government campaigns to encourage HIV or cancer screening tests are another area of public health practice in which ethical principles may conflict. Here again, the goal is to promote the common welfare—for instance, by encouraging individuals to undergo screening tests, although ethical considerations suggest the need to respect the personal autonomy of individuals by not manipulating or coercing them into adopting healthier lifestyles. This requires providing information not only about potential benefits of a screening test, but also about potential risks or harms. The latter information often is provided at the point of screening.

Ethical issues in public health practice are discussed further in Chapter 15, which examines ethical issues raised by AIDS prevention and treatment. A number of ethical conflicts arising in other areas of public health practice are illustrated in the cases that follow.

Case 11a: Ethical Problems Related to Community Concerns Over Contaminated Ground Water

In a semirural community, concern arose over groundwater contamination by an agricultural pesticide that was known to be extremely toxic. Groundwater was the principal source of drinking water for the community. Community residents with contaminated wells were urged not to drink the water.

A well-sampling program was instituted by the local government, with assistance from the federal government, to determine the extent of contamination. Residents were offered access to test results from their own wells and to information about regional patterns of groundwater contamination. The latter involved aggregate data from numerous well tests. Residents (and environmental scientists working on their behalf) were not given access to the individual test results of their neighbors' wells because local government officials felt obligated to protect individual rights to confidentiality. As a result of the lack of specific information about test results from neighborhood wells, it was difficult for residents to determine the likelihood that their own well would become contaminated. This uncertainty was compounded when skepticism arose about the ability of the local government to analyze the data adequately.

Questions for Discussion

1.   Do community residents with contaminated wells have a right to confidentiality? What risks or potential harms might result from release of these data?
2.   Should the environmental scientists who were working on behalf of certain residents of this community have pushed for release of the test data for individual wells, or for greater scrutiny of the local government officials?

Reference

Wartenberg, D. (1996). Ethics in community-based environmental epidemiology and public health practice: Some considerations. *Science of the Total Environment, 184,* 109-112.

Case 11b: Access to Cancer Chemotherapy Protocols by the Elderly

(This case study, which was written by Douglas Weed and Steven Coughlin, is reprinted by permission of Marcel-Dekker, Inc.)

Program planners at a state health department have identified a number of attitudinal, health care system, and knowledge-related barriers that may prevent many older patients with cancer from gaining access to cancer chemotherapy protocols. Many chemotherapy protocols specifically exclude older patients, which has contributed to a lack of information about their effectiveness and potential side effects in this age group. Also, older patients may be reluctant to undergo potentially efficacious therapy because of a lack of knowledge, distrust of physicians, lack of social support, or fatalistic attitudes toward cancer. Community physicians may present therapies unenthusiastically or be unwilling to refer older patients to cancer centers because of concerns about comorbid conditions or toxicity of chemotherapeutic agents in this age group. In addition, less aggressive therapy sometimes has been recommended in the mistaken belief that some tumors, such as breast cancer, are more benign in older patients. Such age-related biases may deter older patients from undergoing state-of-the-art oncological care and result in less favorable prognoses.

In designing a community-based intervention to overcome such barriers, the program planners have discovered that existing resources in the community are insufficient to allow all eligible patients to enroll in potentially lifesaving cancer chemotherapy protocols. Furthermore, they have encountered resistance on the part of community physicians, who feel they are in the best position to make treatment decisions for their patients and, in some instances, fear they will lose patients and potential revenue.

Questions for Discussion

1.   In view of the limited resources, should the program planners target only high-risk or underserved segments of the population, such as older African Americans, or should they seek to improve access to chemotherapy protocols among all older patients?

2.   Should the health department provide referrals and educational materials directly to cancer patients even though some community physicians and hospitals may object?

3.   In considering whether to implement the intervention, the program planners also must consider budgetary constraints. How should they decide between allocating financial resources to the proposed cancer control program and to public health interventions that might benefit other segments of the community, such as programs that address AIDS prevention, infant mortality, or homicide?

References

Weed, D. L. & Coughlin, S. S. (1995). Ethics in cancer prevention and control. In P. Greenwald, B. F. Kramer & D. L. Weed (Eds.), *Cancer prevention and control* (pp. 497-507). New York: Marcel-Dekker.

Hunter, C. P., Frelick, R. W., Feldman, A. R., et al. (1987). Selection factors in clinical trials: Results from the Community Clinical Oncology Program physician's patient log. *Cancer Treat Rep*, 71, 559-565.

Chu, J., Diehr, P., Feigl, P., et al. (1987). The effect of age on the care of women with breast cancer in community hospitals. *J Gerontol*, 42, 185-190.

Case 11c: *Risks and Benefits of Water Chlorination*

A study by governmental researchers in a Latin American country raised questions about the possible risks and benefits of chlorinating the public water supply. Previous efforts to control cholera epidemics had led to the introduction of chlorine as a bactericidal water treatment. Such public health measures had resulted in a decreased incidence of cholera and other diarrheal diseases. The researchers determined that the incidence and prevalence of bladder cancer had increased in the population receiving the chlorinated water over a period of several years. As yet, no studies have been undertaken to determine if the increased risk of bladder cancer is attributable to the consumption of chlorinated water. The contamination of the public water supply by industrial wastes also could account for the excess cases of bladder cancer.

Questions for Discussion

1.   How should risks and potential benefits to the public be balanced in deciding whether to continue chlorination of the water supply in this community?

2.   What should be the investigators' role in helping to formulate such public policies about chlorination of the water supply?

Case 11d: Government Program to Control Mosquito Vectors for Malaria

Malaria is an endemic disease common to many areas of Africa. The bloodborne parasite that causes malaria, *Plasmodium falciparum*, is transferred from the infected host to an uninfected host by means of the *Anopheles* mosquito. The mosquitoes breed easily on stagnant water.

A government program was initiated in one African country to control the mosquito vector by introducing pesticides into water sources that could serve as mosquito breeding grounds. Although the program was successful in helping to control the mosquito population, pregnant women and breastfeeding women were consuming the pesticide-contaminated water, which endangered both their own health and that of their children. Some women were making up infant formula with the contaminated water. Conflicts arose between the need to control malaria transmission and to prevent maternal and child consumption of pesticide-contaminated water.

Questions for Discussion

1. Should the government officials discontinue the pesticide program or continue it?
2. What additional information might they need to reach a decision?

Suggestions for Further Reading

Hahn, R. A. (1994). Ethical issues. In S. M. Teutsch & R. E. Churchill (Eds.), *Principles and practice of public health surveillance* (pp. 175-189). New York: Oxford University Press.

Lappé, M. (1986). Ethics and public health. In J. M. Last (Ed.), *Maxcy-Rosenau's public health and preventive medicine,* (12th Ed., pp. 1867-1877). Norwalk, CT: Appleton-Century-Crofts.

Richards, E. P. & Bross, D. C. (1992). Legal aspects of STD control: public duties and private rights. In K. K. Holmes, P. A. Mardh, P. F. Sparling & P. J. Wiesner (Eds.). *Sexually transmitted diseases,* (2nd Ed.). New York: McGraw-Hill.

Teutsch, S., Berkelman, R. L., Toomey, K. E. & Vogt, R. L. (1991). Reporting for disease control activities. *Am J Public Health, 81,* 932

Vogt, R. L. (1989, July 17–19). Confidentiality: Perspectives from a state epidemiologist. In *Challenge for public health statistics in the 1990s*. Proceedings of the 1989 Public Health Conference on Records and Statistics, National Center for Health Statistics, Washington, DC.

Chapter 12

Studies of Vulnerable Populations

M any public health studies and interventions target vulnerable groups such as children, pregnant women, the elderly, persons with diminished mental capacity, and institutionalized persons. Members of these groups are considered vulnerable because of an increased potential for risks or harms or a decreased capacity for understanding. Understanding the risks and potential benefits of an intervention is an essential element of informed-consent requirements (see Chapter 3), so treatment of those groups raises a number of ethical issues.

Children need parental consent for most research-oriented activities and are usually considered minors until the age of 18. The traditional advocates and decision makers for children are parents (Leikin, 1996). Nevertheless, the autonomy of all potential research participants must be respected, and assent is usually required for children aged 7 years and older.

It sometimes has been argued that research involving children is ethically not permissible if it does not directly benefit the individual child. For example, it has been argued that because children are not capable of giving informed consent, no research ought to be performed on children unless there is the possibility of direct benefit (Ramsey, 1977). Others have convincingly argued, however, that children should be allowed to participate in research, even if they do not stand to benefit directly, provided the research poses no or only minimal risk and parental permission is obtained. In deciding whether to allow children to be included in research studies, researchers must consider not only the risks, but also the negative consequences of not conducting research on children (Leikin, 1996).

In studies of older persons, ethical issues related to informed consent often take on greater significance. Although persons with diminished autonomy are entitled to special protections, such as the requirement that researchers obtain surrogate consent from a close relative of the participant, the need for personal autonomy does not diminish with advancing years.

Minority groups and indigenous populations also may be considered to be at increased risk or otherwise vulnerable. Minority groups are readily identifiable subsets of the population that can be distinguished by racial, ethnic, or cultural heritage. Within such minority groups, subpopulations with unique geographic or national origins and important cultural differences often exist. Other vulnerable groups include individuals who are socioeconomically disadvantaged or marginalized. Such persons may be more motivated to participate in research studies as a result of manipulative or coercive incentives.

A variety of ethical issues that arise in studies of vulnerable populations are highlighted in the cases presented below.

References

Council for International Organizations of Medical Sciences (1993). *International ethical guidelines for biomedical research involving human subjects.* Geneva: CIOMS, 63.

Leikin, S. (1996). Ethical issues in epidemiologic research with children. In S. S. Coughlin & T. L. Beauchamp (Eds.), *Ethics and epidemiology.* (pp. 199-218). New York: Oxford University Press.

Ramsey, P. (1977). Children as research subjects: A reply. *Hastings Center Rep, 7,* 40-42.

Case 12a: The Tuskegee Syphilis Study

The U.S. Public Health Service (PHS) initiated a study in Macon County Alabama in 1932 to examine the natural history of untreated, latent syphilis in Black males. The study included 400 syphilitic men and a comparison group of 200 uninfected men. The participants were not offered antibiotic therapy when penicillin became available in the 1950s, and on several occasions PHS researchers actively sought to prevent treatment.

Scientific reports of the study appeared in the literature every few years beginning in 1936 and continuing through the 1960s. The study was widely reported for years without any significant protest from the medical or scientific communities.

In 1972, when accounts of the study first appeared in the popular media, PHS finally halted the study. At that time, 74 of the participants were still alive. At least 28 of the men (and possibly as many as 100) had died from advanced syphilis.

Questions for Discussion

1.   What questions do cases such as the Tuskegee Syphilis Study raise about the ability of the medical and scientific communities to be self-regulating?

2.   What are the responsibilities of researchers to their study participants? Do researchers have special obligations when the participants are members of vulnerable groups in society or socioeconomically disadvantaged?

References

Brandt, A. M. (1978). Racism and research: The case of the Tuskegee Syphilis Study. *Hastings Center Rep*, 8, 21-29.

Final Report of the Tuskegee Syphilis Study Ad Hoc Advisory Panel, Department of Health, Education, and Welfare. (1973). Washington, DC: U.S. Government Printing Office.

Case 12b: Psychological Risks Posed by Interviewing Procedures

In a case-control study of sudden infant death syndrome in two counties in Great Britain, the parents of deceased infants were interviewed within 72 hours of the infant's death, most within 24 hours. The parents were interviewed about social factors; family history; maternal medical history; details of the pregnancy and perinatal period; and the infant's medical history, including recent signs of illness, feeding, precise details of the infant's last sleep, the position in which he or she had been found, the precise quantity and nature of the clothing and bedding, whether the baby had been swaddled, whether the bedclothes had been over the baby's head when found, what heating was in the baby's room, and how long the heat had been on.

The investigators did not indicate whether any of the parents experienced psychological distress as a result of participating in the study. The study design was methodologically advantageous because the reliability and validity of some information obtained from next-of-kin is likely to decline over time. Other case-control studies of sudden infant death syndrome, however, have examined similar associations while delaying interviews of bereaved parents until six weeks after their baby's death. Prospective studies of high-risk infants, which avoid the need to interview recently bereaved parents, also have been undertaken.

Questions for Discussion

1   To what extent do recently bereaved individuals and other vulnerable populations deserve protective measures—such as measures to ensure that epidemiologic data are obtained in a manner that is not intrusive?
2.   How should obligations not to impair health or cause mental distress be balanced against the need to promote the common good? To what extent should the potential societal benefits of the study be taken into account?

References

Coughlin, S. S. (1996). Ethically optimized study designs in epidemiology. In S. S. Coughlin & T. L. Beauchamp (Eds.), *Ethics and epidemiology* (pp. 145-155) New York: Oxford University Press.

Fleming, P. J., Gilbert, R., Azaz, Y., et al. (1990). Interaction between bedding and sleeping position in the sudden infant death syndrome: A population-based case-control study. *BMJ*, 301, 85-89.

Case 12c: Cancer Control Interventions Aimed at Children

(This case study, which was written by Douglas Weed and Steven Coughlin, is reprinted by permission of Marcel-Dekker, Inc.)

A group of behavioral scientists at an academic research institution plans to design and implement a school-based smoking prevention program in an urban school district. The rationale for the study is based on the observations that cigarette smoking often begins during adolescence and that fewer than one-third of smokers successfully quit once the habit is established. Furthermore, cigarette smoking increases fivefold between the seventh and ninth grades, and 25 percent of 18-year-olds are regular smokers. Overall, cigarette smoking is the most important modifiable factor contributing to premature death and disability in the United States.

The investigators propose to examine the effectiveness of the teacher-delivered educational intervention using a prospective, randomized, controlled design. The participants will consist of several hundred fourth and fifth graders who attend a stratified random sample of inner-city schools. The theoretical framework for the intervention is based on the health belief model and social learning theory. Self-reported information about cigarette smoking will be validated by determining individual levels of serum thiocyanate.

Questions for Discussion

1.   Will the research participants be exposed to any potential risks? If so, do the potential benefits of the study outweigh these risks?

2.   Is it ethical to deny the possible benefits of the educational intervention to children who are randomly allocated to the control group?

3.   What procedures for obtaining the informed consent of the research participants would be desirable?

References

Weed, D. L. & Coughlin, S. S. (1995). Ethics in cancer prevention and control. In P. Greenwald, B. F. Kramer & D. L. Weed (Eds.), *Cancer prevention and control.* (pp. 497-507). New York: Marcel-Dekker.

Walter, H. J., Vaughn, R. D. & Wynder, E. L.(1989). Primary prevention of cancer among children: Changes in cigarette smoking and diet after six years of intervention. *J Natl Cancer Inst,* 81,995-999.

Case 12d: Study of Air Pollution and Asthma in African-American Children

A study was undertaken by a team of government investigators and government contractors to examine the relationship between air pollution and asthmatic symptoms in African-American children. Other stakeholders in the project included the clinics, hospitals, and communities from which the participants were to be recruited. Although the protocol for the 3-year project originally included a beneficial intervention, the team leaders decided to abandon this idea and to use all of the allotted funds to expand the observational pilot study. Many of the community clinics, including those serving low-income populations, had agreed to participate because of the originally planned intervention. A beneficial intervention had been specifically promised by the investigators in order to secure the participation of several of the clinics. Although the situation was not resolved, one investigator did attempt to obtain additional funds that would have made a community-based intervention possible for the low-income clinics.

Questions for Discussion

1.   What are the obligations of investigators to collaborating clinics and other community organizations? When a study is in the planning stages, should the investigators advise the collaborating centers that changes in the study design may take place at a later date?

2.   What are the obligations of researchers to individual participants and to communities in terms of maximizing the potential benefits of public health studies and community interventions?

Suggestions for Further Reading

American College of Physicians. (1989). Cognitively impaired subjects. *Ann Int Med*, 111, 843-848.

Annas, G. & Glantz, L. (1986). Rules for research in nursing homes. *N Engl J Med*, 315, 1157-1158.

Butler, R. (1980). Protection of elderly research subjects. *Clin Res*, 28, 3-5.

Department of Health and Human Services. (1983, March 8). Additional protections for children involved as subjects in research. *Federal Register 48* (46), 9814-9820.

Fulford, K. W. M. & Howse, K. (1993). Ethics of research with psychiatric patients: principles, problems and the primary responsibilities of researchers. *J Med Ethics*, 19, 85-91.

Grodin, M. & Alpert, J. J. (1988). Children as participants in medical research. *Ped Clinics North America*, 35, 1389-1401.

Grodin, M. A. & Glantz, L. H.(1994). *Children as research subjects*. New York: Oxford University Press.

Johns, J. H. (1993). *Bad blood: The Tuskegee Syphilis Experiment*. New York: The Free Press.

Lane, L., Cassel, C. & Bennett, W. (1990). Ethical aspects of research involving elderly subjects: Are we doing more than we say? *J Clin Ethics*, 1, 278-286.

Melnick, V., Dubler, N., Weisbard, A. & Butler, R. (1984). Clinical research in senile dementia of the Alzheimer type: Suggested guidelines addressing the ethical and legal issues. *J Am Geriatrics Soc*, 32, 531-536.

National Commission for the Protection of Human Subjects of Biomedical and Behavioral Research. (1977). Research involving children: report and recommendations. Washington, D.C.: Department of Health, Education, and Welfare Pub. No. (OS) 77-0004 (Appendix), DHEW Pub. No. (OS) 77-0005.

Nolan, K. (1989). Ethical issues in caring for pregnant women and newborns at risk for human immunodeficiency virus infection. *Sem Perinatol*, 13, 55-65.

Ostfeld, A. (1980). Older research subjects: Not homogeneous, not especially vulnerable. *IRB*, 2, 7-8.

Pizzo, P. (1990). Pediatric AIDS: problems within problems. *J Infect Dis*, 61, 316-325.

Ratzan, R. (1980). 'Being Old Makes You Different': The ethics of research with elderly subjects. *Hastings Center Rep*, 10, 32-42.

Reich, W. (1978). Ethical issues related to research involving elderly subjects. *The Gerontologist*, 18, 326-337.

Rothman, D. J. (1982). Were Tuskegee and Willowbrook "studies in nature"? *Hastings Center Rep*, 12, 5-7.

Sachs, G. A. & Cassel, C .K. (1990). Biomedical research involving older human subjects. *Law Med Health Care*, 18, 234-243.

U.S. National Institute on Aging. (1977). Protection of elderly research subjects: Summary of a conference. DHEW Publication No. (NIH) 79-1801. Conference held at the National Institutes of Health in Bethesda, MD, on July 18-19, 1977. Bethesda, MD: U.S. National Institutes of Health.

Chapter 13

Cross-Cultural Research

A culturally sensitive, principled approach to cross-cultural research is needed to ensure that the welfare and rights of participants are protected and that potential benefits to individuals and communities are maximized. The ethical principle of autonomy or self-determination, underlies provisions for obtaining the informed consent of participants in cross-cultural studies and for avoiding excessive incentives that may be manipulative or coercive. These professional obligations are highlighted in a number of international codes of professional conduct for health researchers.

There has been ongoing debate over the transcultural applicability of standards for informed consent and other ethical precepts that have become widely accepted in the United States and Europe. Relativists argue that culturally sensitive standards are needed for obtaining the informed consent of research participants when studies are undertaken in other societies. Others point out the need for some minimal set of universally applicable safeguards that protect the welfare and rights of individuals targeted by health research, as when researchers from the West undertake studies in less developed countries.

In some cultures, it may be necessary to obtain the consent and cooperation of community leaders or heads of households, although this should not replace the requirement of obtaining the informed consent of each individual participant. Provisions for obtaining informed consent in cross-cultural studies may be complicated by language barriers and cultural differences, but persons in other cultures do not as a general rule have diminished capacities for understanding consent requirements.

Researchers also have obligations to balance benefits against risks when carrying out studies in other cultures. Such studies can pose potential risks to groups of individuals and communities.

For example, populations defined by race or ethnicity may suffer stigmatization or lowered self-image following the publication and dissemination of research findings that create or reinforce negative cultural stereotypes. Disparaging information about a group can result in harms such as discrimination in employment, housing, and insurance, or in lowered self-esteem and racial or cultural pride. On the other hand, the identification of disparities in health or the maldistribution of health services across groups defined by race, ethnicity, or lifestyle can serve as a basis for health planning and policy making and thereby contribute to improving the health of those who are less well-off in society.

In cross-cultural studies that rely upon interview data or existing records, there are no physical risks to the participants. Some emotional distress may be experienced, however, as a result of fear of illness, embarrassment, or concerns over violations of privacy. Dimensions of privacy include the sensitivity of the information and the setting being observed (Glanz et al., 1996). Social and legal risks that could result from the disclosure of confidential information should be eliminated or minimized.

Cross-cultural research methods that involve greater community participation and collaboration are more likely to provide long-term benefits to research participants and to the community (Glanz et al., 1996). Potential benefits are more likely to be maximized by participatory research that is collaborative and empowering. Participatory research, which sometimes has been referred to as *action research*, is an interactive learning process that is more likely to develop competencies in the community. Thus, ethical considerations suggest the need for greater participation of research participants in the planning and implementation of cross-cultural studies.

These and other ethical dilemmas arising in cross-cultural studies are illustrated by the case studies that follow.

Reference

Glanz, K., Rimer, B. K. & Lerman, C. (1996). Ethical issues in the design and conduct of community-based intervention studies. In S. S. Coughlin & T. L. Beauchamp (Eds.), *Ethics and epidemiology.* (pp. 156-177). New York: Oxford University Press.

Case 13a: Study of Sexually Transmitted Diseases in a Peri-urban Slum

(This case study, from course materials developed by Gina Etheredge, is included here in revised form with the permission of the author.)

In 1993 researchers from the United States initiated a study in a Caribbean nation to examine sexually transmitted diseases (STDs) in a peri-urban slum. The study protocol was approved by the U.S. investigators' home institution and by the group that sponsored the research in its health clinics. The objectives of the research were to determine the prevalence of four STDs (gonorrhea, chlamydia, syphilis, and trichomoniasis) among childbearing women, to examine risk factors for these infections, and to study the health worker referral system.

The researchers recruited 1,000 pregnant women from the health clinic at the time they presented for their first prenatal check-up. When the women were asked if they would like to participate in the research study, it was explained to them that they would receive a free gynecological examination and that any STDs found would be treated. Such examinations were not routinely available to women residing in this profoundly poor community unless they were already in their third trimester.

Each participant was asked to return for her results 10 days after her initial visit. If a woman tested positive for any STD, she was told by the attending nurse that she must notify her partner or partners who should then report to the clinic for treatment within 5 days. If a partner identified by the research participant did not present at the clinic within 5 days, his name was given by the investigators to the local health worker in charge of the district where the woman resided. The health worker was asked to find this person and to refer him to the physician at the clinic.

Sexual partners of the women who were treated at the clinic were randomized to one of two treatment options. Half of the male partners received free treatment at the clinic; the remainder were given a prescription and asked to go to a community pharmacy to have the prescription filled. The purpose of this randomization was to determine if having to pay for treatment affected completion of therapy.

Questions for Discussion

1.   What ethical concerns does the study raise, if any, in view of the fact that the poor women included in this study did not otherwise have access to gynecological examinations?

2.   Were the researchers justified in releasing the names of the women's sexual partners to local health workers for partner notification?

3.   Are additional ethical issues raised by the randomized study of male partners of the women?

Case 13b: Ethical Problems Surrounding an HIV Vaccine Trial in Africa

A group of French and Zairian scientists published a report in *Nature* on March 19, 1987, stating that one of the investigators, Dr. Daniel Zagury of the Pierrre and Marie Curie University in Paris, had immunized himself with an investigational AIDS vaccine. The researchers also immunized "a small group of Zairians, all of whom were HIV-seronegative and immunologically normal." (Zagury et al., 1987: 249). The trial had received the support of the Zairian Ethics Committee.

This first trial of an AIDS vaccine raised concerns over the possibility that Africans might serve as "guinea pigs" for clinical trials whose conduct would not be permitted in the United States or Europe on ethical grounds. Africans expressed concern that Western investigators might conduct unsupervised "savage experiments." *The New York Times* reported that an unidentified source close to the Zagury group admitted that a major reason they conducted the trial in Zaire was that "It was easier to get official permission [in Zaire] than in France."

Questions for Discussion

1.   What safeguards are needed to protect the rights and welfare of research participants in less developed countries?

2.   Whose ethical standards should be applied to an international vaccine trial such as this one: Those of the researchers' home country (in this case, France) or those of the host country?

References

Christakis, N. A. (1988). The ethical design of an AIDS vaccine trial in Africa. *Hastings Center Rep, 18*, 31-37.

"Zaire, ending secrecy, attacks AIDS openly." (1987, February 8). *The New York Times.*

Zagury, D., Leonard, R., Fouchard, M., et al. (1987). Immunization against AIDS in humans [letter]. *Nature, 326*, 249-250.

Case 13c: Cancer Control Study of Native American Women

A group of cancer control researchers plan to undertake a cross-cultural study of barriers to breast and cervical cancer screening among Native American women in an isolated region of the United States. The aims of the study are to characterize the prevalence and frequency of preventive behaviors and risk factors for cancer in this community, and to identify barriers to breast and cervical cancer screening. It is likely that members of this Native American population encounter substantial barriers to cancer screening because of geographical isolation, rural residence, lack of transportation, poverty, unemployment, lack of education, language barriers, lack of access to health care services, and cultural and attitudinal factors. The research is intended to provide background information needed to design and evaluate future community outreach educational programs aimed at increasing cancer screening in this underserved population.

In planning the study, the researchers carried out in-depth interviews of Native American women and local physicians. Focus-group sessions with about 10 Native American women from the target population are planned to assist with the development of the questionnaire.

A cross-sectional survey of Native American women who are at least 18 years of age is also planned. A structured questionnaire will be developed for use in identifying barriers to breast and cervical cancer screening in this population. A mailing list of heads of households maintained by the Tribal Council will be used to sample the potential respondents. The telephone or in-person interviews will be conducted by trained Native American women research assistants.

The interview form will include questions about demographic and socioeconomic characteristics, general health status, cigarette smoking and use of smokeless tobacco, alcohol consumption, personal and family history of cancer, screening mammography, clinical breast exams, Pap smears, colorectal cancer screening, health care utilization, access to health care, and health priorities for the community. With qualitative information obtained from the focus group sessions as a guide, detailed questions will be included about a number of potential barriers to breast and cervical cancer screening, including behavioral factors, cultural factors, attitudinal factors, and health care system problems faced by the Native American women. The questions will address the extent to which lack of transportation and geographical distance from cancer screening sites prevent the women from obtaining mammograms and Pap smears, as well as fatalistic attitudes about cancer. Additional questions will cover daily life concerns, perceptions about the value of health and about the value of taking specific actions to protect health, perceptions about the quality and availability of preventive care, and knowledge and attitudes about cancer and cancer screening.

The researchers are aware that, many Native Americans differ from the Western perspective in understanding health as a balance between the individual and nature. Illness represents a physical and spiritual disturbance of that balance. The traditional Native American orientation toward life attends to the present rather than the future, and immediate needs are to be dealt with first. Moreover, the group and the extended family are emphasized.

Questions for Discussion

1.   What are the potential risks and benefits of the study to the members of the Native American community?

2.   How can potential risks or harms be minimized in carrying out the research?

3.   How can potential benefits to the Native American community be maximized by the researchers?

4.   What provisions for obtaining the informed consent of the participants would be helpful?

5.   Does the choice of this study population raise any special issues related to equity or justice?

Reference

Michielutte, R., Sharp, P. C., Dignan, M. B., et al. (1994). Cultural issues in the development of cancer control programs for American Indian populations. *J Health Care for the Poor and Underserved*, 5, 280-296.

Suggestions for Further Reading

Angell, M. (1988). Ethical imperialism? Ethics in international collaborative clinical research [Editorial]. *N Engl J Med*, 319, 1081-1083.

Ajayi, O. O. (1980). Taboos and clinical research in West Africa. *J Med Ethics*, 6, 61-63.

Christakis, N. A. (1992). Ethics are local: Engaging cross-cultural variation in the ethics of clinical research. *Soc Sci Med*, 35, 1079-1091.

Council for International Organizations of Medical Sciences. (1993). *International ethical guidelines for biomedical research involving human subjects*. Geneva: CIOMS, 63.

Council for International Organizations of Medical Sciences (1991). *International guidelines for ethical review of epidemiological studies*. Geneva: CIOMS, 31.

De Craemer, W. (1983). A cross-cultural perspective on personhood. *Milbank Q*, 61, 19-34.

Ekunwe, E. O. & Kessel, R. (1984). Informed consent in the developing world. *Hastings Center Rep*, 14, 22-24.

IJsselmuiden, C. B. & Faden, R. R. (1992). Research and informed consent in Africa—Another look. *N Engl J Med*, 326, 830-834.

Kunstadter, P. (1980). Medical ethics in cross-cultural and multi-cultural perspectives. *Soc Sci Med*, 14b, 289-296.

Hall, A. J. (1989). Public health trials in West Africa: Logistics and ethics. *IRB*, 11, 8-10.

LaVertu, D. S. & Linares, A. M. (1990). Ethical principles of biomedical research on human subjects: Their application and limitations in Latin America and the Caribbean. *Bulletin of Pan American Health Organization*, 24, 469-479.

Levine, R. J. (1991). Informed consent: Some challenges to the universal validity of the Western model. *Law Med Health Care*, 19, 207-213.

Olweny, C. (1994). The ethics and conduct of cross-cultural research in developing countries. *Psycho-Oncology*, 3, 11-20.

Schoepf, B. G. (1991). Ethical, methodological and political issues of AIDS research in Central Africa. *Soc Sci Med*, 33, 749-763.

Chapter 14

Genetic Research and Testing

Public health researchers and policy makers are increasingly facing difficult ethical issues relating to the use of genetic testing and screening. Issues include concern over the possibility of discrimination based on an individual's genotype or carrier status, the disclosure of test results to relatives or to other third parties, and the adequacy of informed consent for genetic research on stored tissue samples.

Genetic screening is in part the systematic search in a population for persons with specific genotypes or susceptibilities to environmental agents. Genetic testing and screening may be conducted for research purposes or as part of disease prevention programs. Individuals are detected who are at risk for genetic disease or whose offspring are at risk. Newborn screening, which attempts to identify disease in the newborn, is the most commonly practiced form of genetic screening.

Several instances have been reported in which genetic testing has led to discrimination. State and federal laws such as the Americans with Disabilities Act (ADA) of 1990 may afford some protection against the discriminatory use of genetic tests by employers and insurance companies. Additional legislation, regulatory protections, and strict confidentiality safeguards are needed to minimize risks and potential harms from the release of genetic information to third parties. Informed consent is generally viewed as a requirement for genetic screening and testing.

Screening programs should be conducted only when voluntary testing is shown to be inadequate for preventing serious harm to vulnerable groups.

Special ethical concerns are raised by programs that screen for diseases that occur with increased frequency in specific ethnic and racial groups, such as sickle-cell disease, Tay-Sachs disease, and thalassemia. Sickle-cell screening programs initiated in the United States in the 1960s were politically charged and complicated by insufficient attention to confidentiality and the need for counseling of individuals who tested positive. Some individuals who were found to carry the sickle-cell trait were discriminated against by potential employers or insurance companies.

Genetic testing and monitoring in the workplace also raise questions concerning confidentiality and the control, collection, and dissemination of genetic information. Workplace genetic testing is carried out for a variety of reasons, including research, diagnosis, and the exclusion of workers who are more susceptible to environmentally induced disease. Workers who are asked to undergo such screening may be concerned about possible discrimination or loss of livelihood. They also may fear violations of privacy or the release of confidential information to third parties.

Other ethical issues raised by genetic testing relate to the notification of research participants about their own risks of disease. Knowledge of genetic predisposition to a disease or the determination of carrier status may lead to feelings of inadequacy, fear, or depression and may impair psychological health. Individuals often have difficulty in grasping concepts of risk and probability and may not fully understand the genetic information provided to them.

In recent years, remarkable advances in the field of human genetics and important developments in related fields, such as molecular epidemiology, have given rise to ethical problems that require careful analysis and sound judgment. Some of these problems are highlighted in the cases presented in this chapter.

References

Kenen, R. H. & Schmidt, R. M. (1978). Stigmatization of carrier status: Social implications of heterozygote genetic screening programs. *Am J Public Health*, 68, 1116-1120.

Natowicz, M. R., Alper, J. K. & Alper, J. S. (1992). Genetic discrimination and the law. *Am J Hum Genet*, 50, 465-475.

Rowley, P. T. (1984). Genetic screening: Marvel or menace? *Science*, 225, 138-144.

Case 14a: Screening for Genetic Markers of Cancer Risk

(This case study, which was written by Douglas Weed and Steven Coughlin, is reprinted by permission of Marcel-Dekker, Inc.)

A pediatric oncologist at a regional cancer center has been asked by the mother of a child with childhood sarcoma to screen other members of the family, who range in age from 5 to 45 years of age, for the germ line *p53* mutation that has been associated with the Li-Fraumeni syndrome. This autosomal dominant disorder predisposes people to several forms of cancer, including childhood soft-tissue sarcomas, osteosarcomas and premenopausal breast cancer. Although screening tests for the *p53* mutation may yield false-positive and false-negative results, the predictive power is greatly increased when high-risk populations are screened.

Children from high-risk families who develop brain tumors or sarcomas may have an improved prognosis if the tumor is detected early. Another possible benefit of screening for the *p53* mutation is relief from anxiety among individuals who test negative. However, the risks associated with genetic testing include potential economic losses, discrimination by insurance companies, and adverse psychological effects.

Questions for Discussion

1. Should the oncologist offer the test to the members of this family?
2. What steps should be taken to protect family members from potential discrimination by insurance companies or future employers and from adverse psychological effects?
3. Should the mother have the right to provide proxy informed consent for her underage children?
4. Should the oncologist inform the children about the test results and attempt to explain their significance?

References

Weed, D. L. & Coughlin, S. S. (1995). Ethics in cancer prevention and control. In P. Greenwald, B. F. Kramer & D. L. Weed, (Eds.). *Cancer prevention and control* (pp. 497-507). New York: Marcel-Dekker.

Case 14b: Genetic Screening for BRCA1 and BRCA2 Breast Cancer Genes in Women

A group of cancer control researchers at a state health department and two local universities met to discuss the feasibility and desirability of undertaking a genetic screening study to determine the prevalence of the BRCA1 and BRCA2 breast cancer gene mutations among women in their area. The planning meeting was prompted by the researchers' own varied interests, and by inquiries from local breast cancer advocacy groups following media coverage of cancer susceptibility testing in other groups of women in the United States.

Although BRCA1 and BRCA2 gene mutations have been linked to increased susceptibility to breast and ovarian cancer, more than 100 variants of BRCA1 and several variants of BRCA2 have been identified (Hubbard and Lewontin, 1996). Adequate knowledge of the correct interpretation of these variants is lacking; most of them have not been shown to be associated with tumor growth.

> It is not clear what a women should do if she tests positive [to a variant of BRCA1 or BRCA2], whatever her family history, since there are no effective measures of prevention. 'Early detection' is problematic because it is uncertain what is actually being detected, and even such extreme measures as 'prophylactic' bilateral mastectomy and oophorectomy provide no assurance that a tumor will not develop in the residual tissue (Hubbard and Lewontin, 1996).

Given this uncertainty, it is difficult to know how to counsel women who undergo testing for cancer-associated variants of BRCA1 or BRCA2.

In a series of telephone calls leading up to the planning meeting, the researchers discussed various scientific issues, as well as the ethical and policy issues associated with undertaking a genetic screening study to determine the prevalence of the BRCA1 and BRCA2 breast cancer genes among local women. One member of the research group argued, from "a public health perspective," that the focus of the cancer control research group should be on encouraging women to undergo mammographies (an intervention of known utility) and finding out how to over-come barriers to cancer screening in their area, rather than on cancer susceptibility tests of unknown utility for the patient and with an uncertain risk-to-benefit ratio.

Questions for Discussion

1.   What are the potential risks of genetic testing for BRCA1 or BRCA2 mutations in a research study carried out in the general population?
2.   What ethical considerations underlie the choice of a re-search hypothesis and decisions about what research studies to undertake?

Reference

Hubbard, R. & Lewontin, R. C. (1996). Pitfalls of genetic testing. *N Engl J Med*, 334, 1192-1194.

Case 14c: Genetic Screening of Workers

The development of tests for genetic polymorphisms associ-ated with differential susceptibility to environmental exposures has led some to advocate their use in screening "hypersusceptible" workers.

In one mining town where workers were chronically ex-posed to airborne dust particles, an industrial physician sug-gested that the workers be screened for alpha-1-antitrypsin deficiency, so that workers who were more susceptible to dust-related lung damage could be identified and relocated. On learning of this recommendation, company officials insisted that such workers be terminated, so that the company could avoid having to pay compensation for work-related illnesses that might occur in the future.

Questions for Discussion

1.   Did the physician's recommendation protect the interests of the workers or the company?
2.   What potential harms/risks to workers are associated with genetic screening?

3.   To what extent should employers take such differential susceptibility into account in making decisions about job placement and financial compensation?

4.   If the clinical outcome or the prognostic accuracy of a genetic test is unknown or uncertain, should the workers be provided with test results? Who should control access to such information?

Suggestions for Further Reading

Allen, W. & Ostrer, H. (1993). Anticipating unfair uses of genetic information [Editorial]. *Am J Hum Genet, 53,* 16-21.

Alper, J. S. & Natowicz, M. R. (1993). Genetic discrimination and the Public Entities and Public Accommodations Titles of the Americans with Disabilities Act. *Am J Hum Genet, 53,* 26-32.

American College of Medical Genetics Storage of Genetic Materials Committee. (1997). Statement on storage and use of genetic materials. *Am J Hum Genet, 57,* 1499-1500.

Andrews, L. B., Fullarton, J. E., Holtzman, N. A. et al. (1994). *Assessing genetic risks: Implications for health and social policy.* Washington, DC: National Academy Press.

Annas, G. J. & Elias, S. (Eds.). (1992). *Gene mapping: using law and ethics as guides.* New York: Oxford University Press.

Berg, K. (1983). Ethical problems arising from research progress in medical genetics. In K. Berg & K. E. Trany (Eds.). *Research ethics.* New York: Alan R. Liss, Inc., (pp. 261-275).

Billings, P. R., Kohn, M. A., de Cuevas, M., et al. (1992). Discrimination as a consequence of genetic testing. *Am J Hum Genet, 50,* 476-482.

Buckley, Jr., J. J. (1978). *Genetics now: Ethical issues in genetic research.* Washington, DC: University Press of America.

Council on Ethical and Judicial Affairs and American Medical Association. (1991). Use of genetic testing by employers. *JAMA, 266,* 1827-1830.

Durfy, S. J. (1993). Ethics and the human genome project. *Arch Pathol Lab Med, 117,* 466-469.

Fost, N. (1992). Ethical implications of screening asymptomatic individuals. *FASEB J, 6,* 2813-2817.

Frankel, M. S. & Teich, A. (Eds.). *The genetic frontier: Ethics, law, and policy.* Washington, DC: American Association for the Advancement of Science.

Goodman, K. W. (1996). Ethics, genomics and information retrieval. *Comp Biol Med, 26,* 223-229.

Harper, P. S. (1993). Research samples from families with genetic diseases: A proposed code of conduct. *BMJ, 306,* 1391-1394.

Holtzman, N. A. (1992). The diffusion of new genetic tests for predicting disease. *FASEB J, 6,* 2806-2812.

Holtzman, N. A. & Rothstein, M. A. (1992). Eugenics and genetic discrimination. *Am J Hum Genet, 50,* 457-459.

Juengst, E. T. (1991). Priorities in professional ethics and social policy for human genetics [Editorial]. *JAMA, 266,* 1835-1836.

Kevles, D. J. & Hood, L. (Eds.) (1992). *The code of codes: Scientific and social issues in the human genome project.* Cambridge, MA: Harvard University Press.

Knoppers, B. M. & Chadwick, R. (1994). The human genome project: Under an international microscope. *Science, 265,* 2035-2036.

Knoppers, B. M. & Laberge, C. (1989). DNA sampling and informed consent. *CMAJ, 140,* 1023-1028.

Kodish, E., Murray, T. H. & Shurin, S. (1994). Cancer risk research: What should we tell subjects? *Clin Res, 42,* 396-402.

Lerman, C., Rimer, B. K. &, Engstrom, P. F. (1991). Cancer risk notification: Psychosocial and ethical implications. *J Clin Oncol, 9,* 1275-1282.

Li, F. P., Correa, P. & Fraumeni, Jr., J. F. (1991). Testing for germ line *p*53 mutations in cancer families. *Cancer Epidemiol Biomark Prev, 1,* 91-94.

McCarrick, P. M. (1993). Genetic testing and genetic screening. *Kennedy Inst Ethics J, 3,* 333-354.

McEwen, J. E. & Reilly, P. R. (1992). State legislative efforts to regulate use and potential misuse of genetic information. *Am J Hum Genet, 51,* 637-647.

McEwen, J. E., McCarty, K. & Reilly, P. R. (1992). A survey of state insurance commissioners concerning genetic testing and life insurance. *Am J Hum Genet, 51,* 785-792.

Motulsky, A. G. (1983). Impact of genetic manipulation on society and medicine. *Science,* 219, 135-140.

Murray, T. H. (1991). Ethical issues in human genome research. *FASEB J,* 5, 55-60.

Ostrer, H., Allen, W., Crandall, L. A., et al. (1993). Insurance and genetic testing: Where are we now? *Am J Hum Genet,* 52, 565-577.

Reilly, P. (1992). ASHG Statement on Genetics and Privacy: Testimony to the United States Congress. *Am J Hum Genet,* 50, 640-642.

Report of the Committee on the Ethics of Gene Therapy. (1992). *Human Gene Therapy,* 3, 519-523.

Walters, L. (1991). Human gene therapy: Ethics and public policy. *Human Gene Therapy,* 2, 115-122.

Weir, R. F. & Horton, J. R. (1995). DNA banking and informed consent—Part I. *IRB,* 17(4), 1-4.

Weir, R. F. & Horton, J. R. (1995). DNA banking and informed consent—Part II. *IRB,* 17(5-6), 1-8.

Vineis, P. & Schulte, P. A. (1995). Scientific and ethical aspects of genetic screening of workers for cancer risk: The case of the N-acetyltransferase phenotype. *J Clin Epidemiol,* 48, 189-197.

Chapter 15

HIV/AIDS Prevention and Treatment

The HIV/AIDS pandemic has sharpened concerns about privacy and confidentiality protection in public health. Guidelines for confidentiality in research on AIDS were developed early in the epidemic (Bayer et al., 1984). Persons with AIDS feared that information disclosed for research purposes might be used in ways that could be harmful to them.

Individuals who participate in AIDS research studies may be burdened by a loss of privacy (which is the condition of limited access), by time spent completing interviews and undergoing examinations, and, in some instances, by adverse psychological effects such as anxiety and grief. Other risks include stigmatization and loss of employment or insurance resulting from breaches of confidentiality.

Measures that may be taken to protect individual privacy and ensure the confidentiality of health information include keeping records with personal identifiers under lock and key, limiting access to confidential records to selected members of the research team on a need-to-know basis, discarding personal identifiers from data collection forms and computer files whenever feasible, reinforcing the importance of maintaining the confidentiality of health records at the time of orientation and training sessions for study personnel, and preventing data from being published or released in a form that would allow previously undisclosed identifications to occur.

Other ethical concerns relate to blinded HIV antibody seroprevalence studies that serve an important public health purpose. Vigorous debates have occurred over proposals to unblind anonymous seroprevalence studies carried out for epidemiologic purposes. Objections to such proposals include

the fact that unblinding the seroprevalence studies will compromise the scientific validity of the studies, that confidentiality and
privacy may be violated, and that unblinded studies are more
expensive and time consuming. Blinded surveys provide less
biased estimates of HIV prevalence because individuals do not
choose whether or not to participate. In some countries, such as
England and The Netherlands, blinded serological surveys of
adults and children have been very controversial.

Other ethical issues raised by the HIV/AIDS pandemic
relate to HIV antibody screening, reporting, and partner notification. Mandatory screening for antibodies to HIV has been generally opposed, with few exceptions, because voluntary testing is
more likely to lead to desirable changes in behavior and to limit
the transmission of HIV (Gostin and Curran, 1987). Mandatory
testing also would increase the potential for invasion of privacy,
breaches of confidentiality, and discrimination.

Debates over whether HIV antibody testing should be mandatory bring into focus an important ethical dilemma: the need
for public health professionals to balance the obligation to protect confidentiality with the duty to protect third parties from
becoming infected with HIV (Gostin and Curran, 1987). Recently, there has been debate over whether traditional public
health approaches used to prevent other communicable diseases
(e.g. contact tracing) should be used to limit the spread of HIV
infection and AIDS. Such proposals raise concerns about potential breaches of confidentiality, violation of privacy, and discrimination. Contact tracing for HIV infection is impractical for
high-risk populations such as individuals seen at drug treatment
clinics and gay men living in major metropolitan areas.

AIDS cases are reportable in every state in the United States.
Such reporting serves a valid public health purpose. Some states
also have requirements to report positive HIV antibody tests,
which may be less defensible.

Other ethical challenges relate to HIV surveillance and the
identification of infected newborns. Debates about HIV counseling and testing policies for pregnant women and newborns have
taken place in the context of a broader debate about whether
testing should be voluntary with informed consent or legally
required (Levine, 1996). Until recently, the debate has been

resolved in favor of voluntary HIV antibody testing. Analyses of HIV testing policies for pregnant women generally have concluded that voluntary screening with informed consent is most likely to produce the desired effects of education, prevention, and appropriate medical and social service follow-up (Levine, 1996). The Institute of Medicine in the United States concluded that "individuals (or their legally recognized representatives) should have the right to consent to or refuse HIV testing (except when such testing is conducted anonymously for epidemiologic purposes)."

In the case of pregnant women and newborns, however, the consensus is eroding because of new evidence about the benefits of early diagnosis and intervention in pediatric HIV disease and the results of the AIDS Clinical Trial Group Study 076. Recently, professional groups of pediatricians and obstetricians have issued vigorous calls for routine or mandatory screening. Screening of newborns for HIV antibodies identifies potentially infected newborns and cannot definitively identify an infected infant. Moreover, it discloses the mother's HIV status. As Bayer (1994) observed,

> Mandatory screening of children could become justifiable if therapeutic interventions could substantially extend the lives of infected children, because treatment, regardless of parental objectives, would be imperative. By contrast, the mandatory screening of pregnant women is objectionable because mandatory treatment of competent adults is virtually never acceptable.(p. 1224)

Several ethical issues pertaining to AIDS prevention and treatment efforts are illustrated in the case studies that follow.

References

Bayer, R. (1994). Ethical challenges posed by Zidovudine treatment to reduce vertical transmission of HIV. *N Engl J Med, 331,* 1224.

Bayer, R., Levine, C. & Murray, T. H. (1984). Guidelines for confidentiality in research on AIDS. *IRB, 6,* 1-7.

Gostin, L. & Curran, W. J. (1987). AIDS screening, confidentiality, and the duty to warn. *Am J Public Health, 77*, 361-365.

Levine, C. (1996). Ethics and epidemiology in the age of AIDS. In S. S. Coughlin & T. L. Beauchamp (Eds.) *Ethics and epidemiology.* (pp. 239-254). New York: Oxford University Press.

Case 15a: Ethical and Public Policy Issues Surrounding HIV Home Testing

After years of intense debate, the U.S. Food and Drug Administration (FDA) recently approved the use of diagnostic tests that make it possible for individuals to test for human immunodeficiency virus (HIV) antibody (i.e., evidence of infection with HIV) in the privacy of their own homes. The introduction of such test kits (with the provision of telephone counseling services) had generated considerable controversy and debate. Opponents had warned of disastrous effects including adverse changes in the role of health professionals at important steps in the testing process, potential problems surrounding false-positive test results, and fears that telephone counseling would increase the risk of suicide among individuals testing HIV antibody seropositive. The central ethical and policy question for FDA "is whether home-access HIV tests should be licensed, despite the possible risk to some people of serious psychological sequelae" (Bayer et al., 1995).

Questions for Discussion

1.   What are the potential individual and public health benefits of home testing for HIV? What are the risks?
2.   What is the purpose of federal regulations and statutes on prescription drugs and medical devices?
3.   If FDA had failed to license home testing for HIV, would that decision have been overly paternalistic and intrusive?

References

Bayer, R., Stryker, J. & Smith, M. D. (1995). Testing for HIV infection at home. *N Engl J Med, 332*, 1296-1299.

Harris, H. R. (1994, April 9). "Medical groups, AIDS activists reject at-home testing. *The Washington Post*, p. G1.

Case 15b: High Cost of Combination Therapy with Antiretroviral Drugs

At the international AIDS conference held in July 1996 in Vancouver, British Columbia, scientific reports showed that HIV concentration could be reduced through a combination of antiretroviral drugs including a new class of agents known as protease inhibitors. When protease inhibitors were given in combination with one or more of the reverse transcriptase inhibitors (e.g, AZT), they reduced the amount of virus in the patients' blood below detectable levels and kept it there for months. In view of these dramatic results, there is hope that AIDS may soon become a chronic disease, analogous to diabetes mellitus, that is amenable to medical therapy.

Despite the air of optimism, many of the conference participants expressed concern over the wide gulf between those who could afford the new therapies and those who could not. The combined drug therapies for HIV infection were projected to cost up to $20,000 per year in the United States. There was little hope that individuals in the developing world, where AIDS is rapidly spreading, will have access to the promising new combined therapies.

Questions for Discussion

1.   To what extent should poor individuals, including those in the developing world, have access to potentially lifesaving medical therapies that they cannot afford?

2.   Should pharmaceutical companies that develop lifesaving therapies be free to charge as much as the market will bear, or should drug prices be regulated in some way?

References

Dunlap, D. W. (1996 July 15). In the AIDS fight, bells of hope from Vancouver. At a conference, talk of life, not death. *The New York Times*, p. A6.

Drug companies turn aggressive in promoting new drugs for AIDS. (1996 July 5). *The New York Times,* pp. A1, C6.

Case 15c: Trial of AZT in the Prevention of Vertical Transmission of HIV

(This case study, which is from course materials developed by Judith La Rosa, is included here in revised form with the permission of the author.)

A 3-year, $100,000 grant from the National Institute of Allergy and Infectious Diseases was awarded to study the use of AZT in the possible prevention of the vertical transmission of HIV from mother to child during pregnancy. The efficacy of AZT for this purpose had not been conclusively demonstrated at the time of this study, but the drug had shown promising preliminary results in preventing the vertical transmission of HIV.

The proposed study population (which had been approved by the National Institutes of Health) consisted of 250 pregnant women, mostly Latin and African-American women, who were mostly from low-income housing projects. The investigators gained the cooperation of community leaders in supporting the study concept. Convenient clinics were established in the communities, and Spanish-speaking personnel were hired to assist.

Child care centers for children of the research participants were added to the clinic sites, and the participants were reimbursed for transportation costs. An incentive of $100, to be provided in $25 increments at key points in the study, was offered to prospective participants.

Questions for Discussion

1   Was there sufficient scientific evidence to support the enrollment of participants in this study?

2.   Is the monetary incentive provided to these women, in addition to child care and reimbursement for transportation costs, manipulative or coercive?

Suggestions for Further Reading

Bayer, R. (1989). *Private acts, social consequences. AIDS and the politics of public health.* New York: The Free Press.

Bayer, R., Dubler, N. N. & Landesman, S. (1993). The dual epidemics of tuberculosis and AIDS: Ethical and policy issues in screening and treatment. *Am J Public Health, 83,* 649-654.

Bayer, R., Lumey, L. H. & Wan, L. (1991). The American, British and Dutch responses to unlinked anonymous HIV seroprevalence studies: An international comparison. *Law Med Health Care, 19,* 222-230.

Blendon, R. J. & Donelan, K. (1988). Discrimination against people with AIDS. The public's perspective. *N Engl J Med, 319,* 1022-1026.

Bonkovsky, F. O. (1994). Ethical issues in perinatal HIV. *Clinics in Perinatology, 21,* 15-28.

Brandt, A. M. (1988). AIDS in historical perspective: Four lessons from the history of sexually transmitted diseases. *Am J Public Health, 78,* 367-371.

Faden, R. R., Geller, G. & Powers, M. (1991). *AIDS, women, and the next generation.* New York: Oxford University Press.

Fee, E. & Fox, D. M. (Eds.). (1992). *AIDS. The making of a chronic disease.* Berkeley, CA: University of California Press.

Gostin, L. & Curran, W. J. (1987). Legal control measures for AIDS: Reporting requirements, surveillance, quarantine, and the regulation of public meeting places. *Am J Public Health, 77,* 214-218.

Kegeles, S. M., Coates, T. J. Christopher, T. A. & Lazarus, J. L. (1989). Perceptions of AIDS: The continuing saga of AIDS-related stigma. *AIDS, 3*(Suppl. I), S253-S258.

Levine, C. (1991). Children in HIV/AIDS clinical trials. Still vulnerable after all these years. *Law Med Health Care, 19,* 231-237.

Mann, J. M., Tarantola, D. J. M. & Netter, T. W. & (Eds.) (1992). *AIDS in the world.* Cambridge, MA: Harvard University Press.

Nusbaum, N. J. (1989). Public health and the law: HIV antibody status and employment discrimination. *J AIDS, 2,* 103-106.

Ohi, G., Terao, H., Hasegawa, T., et al. (1988). Notification of HIV carriers: Possible effect on uptake of AIDS testing. *Lancet,* 947-949.

Ploughman, P. (Winter 1995/1996). Public policy versus private rights: The medical, social, ethical, and legal implications of the testing of newborns for HIV. *AIDS & Public Policy Journal,* 10, 182-204.

Reamer, F. G. (Ed.). (1991). *AIDS & ethics.* New York: Columbia University Press.

Chapter 16

Allocation of Scarce Resources and Health Care Reform

E thical concerns in public health often relate to the just alloca tion of scarce resources, including health care services. The importance of this topic is indisputable today in this era of budgetary constraints and health care reform. Because of rising health care costs and finite resources, it is impossible to provide every procedure or preventive measure that might possibly benefit every individual and still manage to care for everyone (Smith, 1996).

In managed care, efforts to control costs may conflict with health care providers' obligations to advocate on behalf of patients who need costly services. This tension between doing what is best for the patient and ensuring a just allocation of scarce resources is at the heart of managed care ethics. Whereas physicians have traditionally been guided by principles of autonomy and beneficence in the context of being advocates for their patient, institutions such as health maintenance organizations (HMOs) are guided instead by notions of efficiency, cost-effectiveness, cost reduction, and optimal resource allocation (Perkel, 1996). The challenge is to find an equitable way to distribute health care resources that does not unduly conflict with other ethical principles.

The equitable distribution of goods and services such as health care services is grounded in ethical principles of justice (principles of fairness and equity in the distribution of benefits and risks), as introduced in Chapter 1. Utilitarian theories of justice emphasize a mixture of criteria so that public goods are maximized. But utilitarian approaches can fail to consider adequately the final distribution of benefits (and harms) to small subgroups of the population.

Libertarian theories of justice, on the other hand, emphasize rights to social and economic liberty. These theories hold that distributions of goods and services such as the potential benefits of public health research are best left to the marketplace. Events in a true free market are matters of individual choosing and enterprise rather than matters of social planning by government. Such theories provide little protection for socioeconomically disadvantaged persons in society.

An egalitarian theory of justice implies that each person (or class of persons) in society should share equally in the distribution of potential benefits. A theory of justice proposed by John Rawls holds that society has an obligation to correct inequalities in the distribution of resources. Under this theory, those who are least well-off ought to benefit most from public services such as health care. One of the problems with this theory is that it can lead to a reduction of the resources available to society as a whole, thereby reducing the aggregate benefit of any limited resources. This theory of justice also permits maldistributions of resources that favor the least well-off. Nevertheless, Rawl's theory does provide considerable support for maximizing benefits to socially disadvantaged persons, particularly if it can be demonstrated that aiding those who are least well-off ultimately benefits society as a whole.

Many of these issues related to distributive justice and the allocation of scare public health resources are illustrated by the case studies provided in this chapter. The first case is from the public health and medical discipline of health care administration.

References

Beauchamp, T. L. & Childress, J. F. (1994). *Principles of biomedical ethics* (4th Ed.). New York: Oxford University Press.

Perkel, R. L. (1996). Ethics and managed care. *Med Clinics North Am*, 80, 263-78.

Smith, A. J. K. (1996). Avoiding the ethical pitfalls of managed care. *Minn Med*, 79, 24-26.

Case 16a: HMO Contracts

In the mid-1990s, many patients belonging to for-profit health maintenance organizations (HMOs) began to question the candor of the recommendations they received from their doctors. At that time, many HMO contracts had a clause, referred to by critics as a "gag rule," that forbade physicians from disclosing certain information to their patients, including financial incentives provided by the HMOs to encourage doctors to limit care and reduce costs. Critics charged that many HMOs were offering doctors financial incentives to minimize care and to recommend fewer or less costly treatments to their patients. Nevertheless, managed care, HMOs, and other cost-saving measures may help to bring under control runaway medical costs associated with the fee-for-service approach.

In 1996, the federal government in the United States joined several states in outlawing such gag rules.

Questions for Discussion

1. How could physicians have reconciled "gag rules" contained in some for-profit HMO contracts with their responsibility to always act in the best interests of their individual patients? To what extent did such clauses present conflicting interests?
2. What are the responsibilities of physicians to fully inform their patients about treatment options?

Reference

Gagging the doctors. Critics charge that some HMOs require physicians to withhold vital information from their patients. (1996, January 8) *Time*, p. 50.

Case 16b: Health Care for Undocumented Aliens

In 1994 California voters approved Proposition 187, legislation to restrict or eliminate access by illegal immigrants to a variety of public services, including health care. One provision of the measure requires that health providers and others report suspected illegal aliens to authorities:

If any publicly-funded health care facility in this
state from whom a person seeks health care services,
other than emergency medical care as required by
federal law, determines or reasonably suspects, based
upon the information provided to it, that the person is
an alien in the United States in violation of federal law,
the following shall be followed by the facility: 1) The
facility shall not provide the person with services; 2)
The facility shall, in writing, notify the person of his or
her apparent illegal immigration status, and that the
person must either obtain legal status or leave the
United States; 3) The facility shall also notify the State
Director of Health Services, the Attorney General of
California, and the United States Immigration and
Naturalization Service of the apparent illegal status,
and shall provide any additional information that may
be requested by any other public entity.

After the legislation was passed, there were a number of
reports that illegals were forgoing health care for fear of being
deported. In some cases, according to initial reports, patient loads at
some clinics declined 20 percent. Elsewhere, there were fears of
increases in tuberculosis. A Hospital Council of Southern California
spokesperson called Proposition 187 "a public health nightmare."

Questions for Discussion

1.   Do undocumented aliens have a right to health care? Should
their care be paid for by taxes collected from legal residents of the
United States?
2.   Should health workers be required to turn illegal immigrants over to authorities?
3.   Would it be possible to distinguish, for purposes of public
policy, between communicable diseases and other medical conditions for which illegal aliens might require health care?

References

Aston, G. (1995, January 9). Hospitals join the fight. *American Hospital News*, p. 7.

Ziv, T. A. & Lo, B. (1995). Denial of care to illegal immigrants: Proposition 187 in California. *New Engl J Med*, 332, 1095-1098.

Nickel, J. W. (1986). Should undocumented aliens be entitled to health care? *Hastings Center Rep*, 16, 19-23.

Case 16c: Cancer Screening in Socioeconomically Disadvantaged Populations

(This case study, which was written by Douglas Weed and Steven Coughlin, is reprinted by permission of Marcel-Dekker, Inc.)

A community-based organization that conducts educational outreach programs to encourage individuals to comply with recommended guidelines for cancer screening is concerned that low-income residents may not be benefiting from existing educational programs. Mortality rates for many cancer sites are particularly high among patients of low socioeconomic status, and socioeconomic factors appear to play an important role in cancer stage at diagnosis and survival. Furthermore, lower socioeconomic status—as measured by income, educational level, or employment status—has been associated with noncompliance with recommended guidelines for cancer screening. Structural barriers such as a lack of health insurance or affordable services, lack of transportation or accessibility, and heavy family commitments may prevent many low-income residents from receiving preventive health care. In addition, economically disadvantaged individuals who undergo screening may be less likely to return for follow-up and treatment.

Questions for Discussion

1.   How much of its resources should the organization devote to the prevention and early detection of cancer among the socioeconomically disadvantaged? On what considerations should such decisions be based?

2.   How should the health agency determine whether an educational program or mass media campaign directed at underserved individuals is acceptable to the target population? Is some form of informed consent necessary?

References

Weed, D. L. & Coughlin, S. S. (1995). Ethics in cancer prevention and control. In P. Greenwald, B. F. Kramer & D. L. Weed (Eds.), *Cancer prevention and control.* (pp. 497-507). New York: Marcel-Dekker.

Bloom, J. R., Hayes, W. A., Saunders, F., et al. (1987). Cancer awareness and secondary prevention practices in black Americans: Implications for intervention. *Fam Commun Health,* 10, 19-30.

Denniston, R. W. (1981). Cancer knowledge, attitudes, and practices among black Americans. In C. Mettlin & G. P. Murphy (Eds.). *Cancer among black populations.* (pp. 225-236). New York: Liss.

Freeman, H. P. (1989). Cancer in the socioeconomically disadvantaged. *CA,* 39, 267-288.

Suggestions for Further Reading

Annas, G. J. (1995). Reframing the debate on health care reform by replacing our metaphors. *N Engl J Med,* 332, 744-745.

Bayer, R. (1994). Ethical challenges posed by Zidovudine treatment to reduce vertical transmission of HIV. *N Engl J Med,* 331, 1224.

Fromer, L. M. (1994). Ethics in managed care. *Hospital Practice,* 29, 51-52.

Jecker, N. S. (1995). Business ethics and the ethics of managed care. *Trends Health Care Law Ethics,* 10, 53-55.

Lappé, M. (1986). Ethics and public health. In J. M. Last (Ed.), *Maxcy-Rosenau's public health and preventive pedicine* (12th ed., pp. 1867-1877). Norwalk, CT: Appleton-Century-Crofts.

La Puma, J. (1993). Anticipated changes in the doctor-patient relationship in the managed care and managed competition of the Health Security Act of 1993. *Arch Fam Med,* 3, 665-671.

Macklin, R. (1995). The ethics of managed care. *Trends Health Care Law Ethics,* 10, 63-66.

Morreim, E. H. (1995). *Balancing Act: The new medical ethics of medicine's new economics.* Dordrecht, The Netherlands: Kluwer.

Parish, D. C. (1995). Medical ethics and managed care. *J Med Assoc Georgia,* 84, 171-172.

Pellegrino, E. D. (1994). Ethics. *JAMA,* 271, 1668-1670.

Potter, R. L. (1995). An integrated ethics program for managed care organizations. *Trends Health Care Law Ethics*, 10, 87-90.

Roman, K. M. Medical ethics vs. managed care: Medical journals voice physicians' concerns. *J Arkansas Med Soc*, 92, 125-126.

Thomasma, D. C. (1995). The ethics of managed care and cost control. *Trends in Health Care Law & Ethics*, 10, 33-36.

INSTRUCTOR'S GUIDE

The cases and discussion questions in this book are intended for use in courses on public health ethics in graduate degree programs and continuing professional education programs. They also are suitable for interactive lecture series and workshops on ethics in public health sciences. The cases include many that have never been reported as such, some that are quite well known in human subjects literature (e.g., the Tuskegee syphilis study), and others drawn from current events (e.g., communicating about health risks from "mad cow disease"). Such a mixture seems especially well-suited for courses intended to raise awareness of ethical issues.

On the basis of our own experiences in teaching courses and conducting workshops on public health ethics, we recommend use of the case study approach, in which students are asked to review ethics cases on a particular topic and then come to class prepared to analyze and discuss them. The case study approach works best if a relatively small group of students face each other in round-table fashion.

The role of the discussion leader is to help the students learn how to identify and solve ethical problems and conflicts arising in public health. A combination of lectures and small group discussions of assigned readings and case studies can be used for this purpose. The students also should be exposed to the burgeoning literature on the ethics of public health research and practice; the bibliography provided in this text is a useful starting point.

The topics that can be covered generally follow the chapter outline of this book. These include a framework for ethics in public health, ethics guidelines for public health professionals, privacy and confidentiality protection, issues surrounding informed consent, the ethics of randomized controlled trials, committee review and the institutional review board system in the United States, communication responsibilities of public health professionals, issues surrounding the publication and interpretation of research findings, conflicting interests and the ethics of research sponsorship, and scientific misconduct in public health research. Other topics that can be covered include ethical issues in public health practice, the ethics of cross-cultural research, genetic discrimination, the ethics of AIDS prevention and treatment, and the allocation of scarce resources and health care reform. An important goal of such courses should be to discuss cultural differences and perspectives on ethical issues such as informed consent and to identify issues arising in studies of vulnerable persons such as children, the elderly, and indigenous populations. The case studies and topics for discussion should encompass responsibilities to study participants, responsibilities to society, responsibilities to employers and funding sources, and responsibilities to professional colleagues.

Courses in public health ethics are designed not to improve the moral character of students, but instead to provide them with the conceptual abilities and decision-making skills they will need to deal successfully with ethical issues in the sciences that underlie public health research and practice. In this way, such courses go beyond simply sensitizing students to ethical problems in public health. The cognitive aspects of public health ethics that can be taught using the case study approach include the identification of the ethical commitments of public health research and practice, recognition of ethical issues and problems in public health, critical reflection on one's personal values and obligations as a public health professional, knowledge of central concepts such as the elements of informed consent, understanding of important decision making procedures, and the application of concepts and methods for ethical decision making to actual cases in public health ethics. The latter involves identification of the relevant principles, rules, duties, or obligations; clarification of tensions between principles and the attempt to resolve such tensions through further specification; and making and justifying ethical decisions through moral reasoning. An important part of this process is the identification of possible objections to ethical choices and reasons for such objections, and formulation of counter-arguments or modification of previously reached ethical decisions.

In the discussion that follows, we provide concise analyses of cases presented in the text, analyses we hope will be of use and interest to instructors and students alike.

References

Coughlin, S. S. (1996). Model curricula in public health ethics. *Am J Prev Med*, 12, 247-251.

Culver, C. M., Clouser, K. D., Gert, B., et al. (1985). Basic curricular goals in medical ethics. *New Engl J Med*, 312, 253-256.

Pellegrino, E. D., Siegler, M. & Singer, P. A. (1990). Teaching clinical ethics. *J Clin Ethics*, 1, 175-180.

Chapter 2: Protection of Privacy and Confidentiality

The first case in this chapter, involving confidentiality of information collected from men at increased risk for HIV infection, illustrates some of the confidentiality and consent issues that can arise in HIV/AIDS research. The researchers must balance the need to ensure the confidentiality of the interview information, as promised in the original informed consent statement, with the need to protect those who might have received contaminated blood. In certain situations, autonomy-based obligations to protect the confidentiality of medical information can be validly overridden by other principles and action guides with which they conflict. In the case presented here, the rights and welfare of those who might have received HIV contaminated blood also must be taken into account. It is not enough to consider the rights of the research participants and the obligations of the researchers to rigorously protect the confidentiality of medical information.

In what circumstances would it be permissible for the researchers to violate their pledges of confidentiality? To whom would the information be disclosed and under what conditions? It might be possible to recontact the HIV antibody seropositive individuals who had given blood and ask for their permission to release this information to the Red Cross in order to determine whether or not the blood had been discarded. The confidentiality safeguards employed by the Red Cross then would be of interest.

Researchers also have an obligation to respect the law, and possible courses of action in situations such as this are informed by both case law and federal and state regulations (although these can vary greatly).

Researchers should generally try to anticipate such prob-·
lems before finalizing their interviewing procedures and obtaining the informed consent of participants. This may be easier said
than done, however.

In the second case study, state privacy laws governing
access to medical records, and their strict interpretation by an
Institutional Review Board (IRB), are seen as an obstacle to
epidemiologic research. The role of the IRB is to examine the risks
and benefits of proposed research studies and to ensure that the
provisions for obtaining the informed consent of participants are
adequate. As this case suggests, IRBs also protect the interests of
the institution at which the research is carried out.

Patients have a right to expect that their personal privacy
and the confidentiality of their medical records will be protected.
With few exceptions, their medical records should not be released to a third party unless they have given their informed
consent. However, these rights are not absolute and there are
several situations in which medical records are routinely released to a third party without the informed consent of the
patient (e.g. release of records to quality assurance teams or
qualified health researchers). The ethical implications of not
undertaking the research also must be taken into account; overly
restrictive privacy laws may prevent researchers from gaining
important new insights into disease etiology and prevention. On
balance, it seems reasonable to conclude that the potential benefits of health research to society, to future patients, and to the
community outweighs the need to protect patient confidentiality, especially in those situations in which the potential risks to
patients are minimal, the study protocol has been reviewed by an
IRB, and it is not feasible to obtain the informed consent of
patients before their medical records are reviewed by members
of the research team.

Of course, researchers have a responsibility to ensure that
the confidentiality of personal health information is vigorously
protected. Measures that may be taken to protect individual
privacy and ensure the confidentiality of health information
include keeping personal identifiers under lock and key; limiting
access to confidential records to selected members of the research
team on a need-to-know basis; separating and, in time, discard-

ing personal identifiers from data collection forms and computer files; reinforcing the importance of maintaining the confidentiality of health records at the time of orientation and training sessions for study personnel; and various measures to prevent data from publication or release in a form that would allow breaches of confidentiality to occur.

The third case involves the release of cancer registry data to a third party. Public health researchers must respect that the law and court subpoenas, such as the ones stemming from this court case, are legally binding. The officials at the Illinois Department of Public Health did attempt to inform the court about the obligations of public health professionals to protect the confidentiality of health information, but only some of their recommendations were heeded. Even when personal identifiers such as names and addresses were removed from the records, there was still a potential for breaches of confidentiality through linkages with residential postal codes. Improved legislation is needed to prevent unintended breaches of confidentiality stemming from future cases in which public health officials are required to turn over confidential health information to a third party.

Principles of justice suggest that the children who developed neuroblastoma may be entitled to financial compensation for their illnesses, assuming that the cause of the illnesses can be established. In this case, the right of the neuroblastoma victims to receive compensation for their illnesses must be balanced against the need to protect the confidentiality of the health information collected by the Illinois Department of Public Health. The principle of autonomy underlies such rules of confidentiality.

Chapter 3: Informed Consent in Public Health Research

In the first case in this chapter, the adequacy of informed or valid consent in a seroepidemiologic study of HTLV-II in Panamanian children is examined. Although the researchers obtained the consent of the mothers at the time of the original study of *Toxoplasma gondii*, no information was provided about the risks or potential benefits of the seroepidemiologic study of HTLV-II since that study had not even been envisioned at the time of the original survey. The mothers of the research participants were not told that a duplicate sample of the child's sera would be saved for possible future use.

In general, participants have a right to be informed about the purpose of the research, its scientific methods and procedures, any anticipated risks and benefits, and any anticipated inconveniences or discomfort. Furthermore, they may refuse to participate or withdraw from the research at any time without penalty.

The researchers should make every effort to recontact the participants and their legal guardians to obtain consent before testing the banked sera for antibodies to HTLV-II. If contacting participants or guardians is not possible, then it would be helpful to obtain some other form of informed consent—for example, by contacting representatives of the Indian communities about the study. A further reason for recontacting the original participants is that researchers have an obligation to provide individuals who take part in health research with their test results and to help them interpret those results.

If the researchers cannot recontact the original participants or their guardians, then the question becomes whether the potential benefits of the seroepidemiologic study, both to society at large and to the Native American communities, outweigh the risks. Potential harms and risks to the Native Americans include stigmatization and discrimination, although these are admittedly remote possibilities. The researchers could minimize such risks by carefully explaining their results when communicating them to the scientific community and to the media.

The failure to make the most use of scarce biological specimens also has ethical implications. The commitment of public health researchers to the advancement of knowledge should not outweigh or override all other considerations, however.

The second case involves the intentional nondisclosure of information in a study of cocaine use among minority inner-city clinic patients. As a general rule, researchers are obligated to disclose those facts that participants usually consider salient in deciding whether to consent to a proposed study or procedure. The clinic patients almost certainly would wish to be informed about the testing of their urine for cocaine metabolites, even if they had no reason to believe that they would test positive. If the participants had been fully informed about the study, the response rate would likely have been lower. In designing the study to ensure scientific validity, the investigators failed to respect the participants' right to make informed decisions. Because the study dealt with illicit drug use, which is illegal, the risks to the participants through inadvertent breaches of confidentiality were potentially serious. The fact that body fluids were assayed by the investigators is material, since the invasion of privacy is greater.

The ethics of research involving deception have been extensively debated in the literature, mostly by psychologists and behavioral scientists. Deception is rarely a justifiable research technique; it may, however, be acceptable for addressing research questions that cannot otherwise be answered, provided potential risks are minimal and the protocol has been reviewed by an institutional review board. Nevertheless, deception may reduce trust of investigators in studies of minority communities.

The third case considers the duty of researchers to inform participants in radiation experiments sponsored by the U.S. Government. Even in the name of national security interests, requirements for obtaining the consent of persons who are members of the general public should not be waived. Since the Nuremberg trials, the disclosure of information to patients and research participants has been deemed essential. President Clinton's Advisory Committee on the Human Radiation Experiments recommended that many of the patients exposed to radiation in experiments sponsored by the U.S. Government receive compensation for their injuries.

Chapter 4: Randomized Controlled Trials

The first case in this chapter examines the ethics of randomized controlled trials of bone marrow transplants for the treatment of advanced breast cancer in women. Some ethicists have argued that patients with life-threatening conditions do not have a *right* to receive experimental therapies of unproven effectiveness. Nevertheless, policies that prevent patients from having access to such therapies outside of randomized trials have been criticized as being manipulative or coercive.

The potential risks associated with the widespread adoption of this experimental procedure before it has been adequately tested include possible diminished survival in women with advanced breast cancer, unanticipated side effects, and excessive financial costs to society. On the other hand, the potential benefits include possible improved survival for women who are currently living with advanced breast cancer.

Physicians who receive financial incentives to recruit patients for a clinical trial may encounter a conflict between their own interests and their duties to their patients and to society. Physicians traditionally owe their greatest allegiance to their patients.

The next case deals with an early randomized controlled trial of continuous oxygen administration in premature infants at risk for retrolental fibroplasia. This historical case provides a strong argument in favor of the use of properly designed and conducted randomized trials to evaluate new clinical therapies. For such trials to be ethical, there must be genuine uncertainty about the comparative therapeutic merits of each treatment arm.

The third case in this chapter considers a randomized trial of tamoxifen in the primary prevention of breast cancer. The investigators must minimize risks and maximize potential benefits to the participants and to society. They must consider whether the risks are outweighed by the potential benefits and whether it is ethical to deny possible benefits from the trial to women randomly allocated to the placebo group.

This balancing of risks and potential benefits may be influenced by the choice of study population. For example, the risks may be greater for premenopausal women, for whom less evidence is available from observational studies about the potential side effects of long-term tamoxifen therapy.

In view of the enhanced scientific validity of randomized trials, it might be argued that the most desirable approach would be to carry out the trial expeditiously to maximize benefits for the greatest number of people (a utilitarian perspective). It also might be argued that there is no ethical obligation to provide tamoxifen to high-risk women (such as those randomly allocated to the control group), because its effectiveness in chemoprevention has yet to be demonstrated.

The ethical implications of not conducting a trial of this nature also must be considered. For example, there may be hazards associated with the widespread adoption of a chemopreventive agent that has not been adequately tested.

A further consideration is whether adequate numbers of minority women will be included to ensure that the results are generalizable to them.

Important questions may be asked about the ability of lay persons to understand adequately the risks and potential benefits associated with participation in the trial. As new information about potential side effects becomes available during the course of the trial, it may be necessary to revise the informed consent documents.

Chapter 5: Committee Review and the Institutional Review Board System

The first case in Chapter 5 deals with the multi-institutional review of a research protocol. Institutional review boards weigh the risks and potential benefits of proposed research studies and try to ensure that the procedures for obtaining the informed consent of participants are adequate. They also consider whether the procedures for recruiting study participants will assure an equitable distribution of the risks and potential benefits of the research.

The use of local committees to review research protocols ensures that local customs and normative rules can be taken into account. As this case illustrates, however, the use of local rather than regional or national committee review can result in substantial bureaucratic obstacles to multi-institutional studies. To reduce such problems, local institutional review boards (IRBs) should allow for maximum flexibility in informed consent statements and other procedures.

In the second case, an institutional review board grapples with a retrospective study of clinical test results. It is common for such review committees to require investigators to obtain the approval of each patient's physician before contacting the patient to obtain his or her informed consent. Although such procedures have been criticized as being "paternalistic," they do protect the institution's interests and those of the attending physicians. In some situations, it also may be in the interest of individual patients for their physician to act as a "gatekeeper" in this way.

The use of medical records for health research generally poses only minor risks, provided steps are taken to protect the confidentiality of the records. Although the release of medical records to qualified health researchers does infringe upon patients' rights to privacy, such harms may be greatly outweighed by the potential benefits of the research to society and to future patients. If the patients are to be contacted for some additional form of research, such as a telephone interview, then their informed consent should be requested at the time of the patient contact.

The next case has to do with IRB review of a needle exchange program evaluation study. IRB members who evaluate such studies must weigh risks and potential benefits and determine whether the informed consent procedures are adequate. Of special concern in this evaluation study are the risks to the individuals randomly allocated to the second group. The IRB members must decide whether there will be an equitable distribution of potential benefits from the trial, including a reduced risk of acquiring HIV and other bloodborne pathogens. Many risk reduction programs in public health, such as needle exchanges and condom distribution programs, remain controversial. A consensus about how best to evaluate such programs, or whether to implement them, may not emerge.

Chapter 6: Scientific Misconduct in Public Health Research

The first case in this chapter surrounds the removal of Bernard Fisher as Principal Investigator of the National Surgical Adjuvant Breast and Bowel Project (NSABP). This episode is one of several recent cases involving allegations of misconduct (in Fisher's case, it was actually one of his many co-investigators who had falsified the data) that have been widely covered in the media. Such controversies may lead to situations in which investigators are "tried in the media," as well as to political pressure and calls for funding agencies to take some action. Health researchers are entitled to due process, however, and the rights of the accused must be taken into account. Allegations of misconduct and other serious improprieties require careful investigation and sound judgment. This controversial case illustrates how the whole scientific enterprise can be damaged by incidents of misconduct that lead to loss of public confidence and support.

Principal investigators of multicenter clinical trials and health researchers at coordinating centers have a responsibility to scrutinize data collected by collaborators at participating centers and to otherwise ensure quality control. Standards in the field have improved in recent years as procedures for quality control have been refined. Other responsibilities of clinical trials researchers to the public, to funding agencies, and to professional colleagues are detailed in recently formulated ethics guidelines for epidemiologists and other medical researchers.

The second case deals with allegations of scientific misconduct against an investigator. The allegations were ultimately dismissed. Such cases underscore the need for confidentiality and due process in investigations of possible misconduct. Although reasonable steps should be taken to protect accused investigators from untoward publicity, society's interests and the integrity of the scientific enterprise are protected by vigorous investigations into possible cases of misconduct.

The next case examines the possible violation of professional standards by an environmental scientist. There are many forms of scientific misconduct, only some of which are dealt with by funding agencies and other institutions.

The ethics guidelines that have been proposed for epidemiologists and other health researchers outline responsibilities to professional colleagues (e.g., reporting results and reporting unacceptable behavior and conditions) as well as responsibilities to individual research participants and whole communities (e.g., providing benefits and maintaining public trust). The guidelines do not provide an exhaustive account of the responsibilities of public health professionals, however. In many instances, such as in this case, the best course of action may be difficult to discern.

Conflicts between researchers can be best avoided by formulating the responsibilities each researcher has to other members of the team—in writing, in advance—to make sure that there is a clear understanding of the conditions under which research results will be released to the public and by whom. This is particularly important when the team consists of researchers from several different disciplines and backgrounds.

One notable observation about this case is that the environmental expert who was criticized for a lack of scientific objectivity is a woman. Although gender bias remains pervasive in the scientific community, it is difficult to know whether this problem contributed to the complaints against the environmental expert.

The last case in this chapter relates to the falsification of data from an environmental study. Although instances of data falsification or fabrication are relatively uncommon, investigators need to ensure that their co-investigators are well qualified and that proper data handling procedures are employed. These include routine audits, thorough record keeping, well-maintained laboratory notebooks, and so forth. When instances of possible data tampering come to light, researchers do have an obligation to society and to other members of their profession to confront the individual and, if warranted, to report the incident to the proper institutional body.

Chapter 7: Conflicting Interests and Research Sponsorship

The first case in this chapter relates to concern over microwave exposure at the U.S. Embassy in Moscow. The case illustrates some general principles concerning the obligations of health researchers to study participants and the need to avoid potential conflicting interests.

Health researchers have ethical and professional obligations to minimize risks and maximize potential benefits of research studies, both to participants and to society. These obligations are reflected in ethics guidelines for health researchers. Researchers also have an obligation to respect the autonomy of persons who participate in research studies; this principle underlies rules of disclosure. Research participants have the right to receive relevant information about risks and potential benefits. Disclosure of results refers not only to the overall findings of health studies, but also to each individual's test results.

Health researchers have a further responsibility to choose appropriate study designs and to interpret biological test results correctly. Some perspective on each participant's results should be provided, even if the meaning of the results is incompletely understood.

The second case in this chapter addresses cardiovascular research sponsored by the tobacco industry. Conflicting interests can occur when a public health researcher makes a judgment about the causality of an association while being influenced by financial interests that impair his or her objectivity or impartiality. However, it is necessary to distinguish actual conflicting interests from those that are potential conflicts, as well as from situations in which there is an appearance of conflicting interests. For example, a health researcher who accepts funding from the tobacco industry might appear to have conflicting interests, or at least possible conflicting interests, but more information would be required to know whether a conflict actually exits.

Many universities attempt to prevent conflicts of interest with policies such as those requiring that contracts with research sponsors contain specific clauses permitting researchers to report the results of their research, even if the findings are unfavorable from the standpoint of the sponsor or funding agency. University-based researchers also have certain academic freedom rights, and such rights must be taken into account when institutional policies regarding research funding are developed.

The next case deals with the divulgence of research funding sources. Many leading journals require authors of scientific reports and editorials to divulge their sponsors when articles are submitted for publication. The extent to which such funding sources represent actual conflicting interests often is unclear, however. Although actual and potential conflicting interests must be distinguished, even the appearance of conflicting interests can damage trust or credibility in some situations.

The fourth case relates to conflicting interests in an environmental impact assessment in an African country. This case further illustrates the conflicting interests that can arise in sponsored research, including environmental risk assessments, and the need to avoid being unduly influenced by financial interests that impair objectivity or impartiality. This case also illustrates that officials in developing countries often have perspectives that differ from those of individuals from industrialized nations in terms of public policy priorities. Ethical issues underlie many public policy disputes.

Concern over peer review of government-sponsored research is the focus of the fifth case in this chapter. Both researchers and funding agencies have obligations to identify their respective responsibilities and to protect privileged information. Further obligations are to maintain objectivity and impartiality and to communicate concerns effectively and promptly. Conflicting interests may explain the actions of the government funding agency, but not enough information is available to conclude that an actual conflict exists.

The last case in this chapter has to do with conflicting interests in a study of occupational lung disease. The researchers must balance the need to respect the company's concerns with the need to respect the rights of the workers. Of overriding concern are the welfare of the workers and their right to receive important information that may help them to protect their health. Workers have a right to be informed about the results of the study, including information that may help them to understand their own risk of disease.

Chapter 8: Intellectual Property and Data Sharing

The first case in this chapter involves conflicts between colleagues at a university. By making the data set available to her newly-appointed colleague, the faculty member who completed the initial study increased the potential benefits of the initial data set. There should have been an explicit understanding between the two faculty members, however, about how the data set would be handled and about who would participate in the development of the grant application. Ideally, such agreements should have been documented in writing. There also should have been a written contract detailing responsibilities to the industrial sponsors of the study, such as protecting the confidentiality of the records.

The next case, concern over plagiarism by a department chair, illustrates additional issues having to do with intellectual property rights and scientific misconduct. Issues that determine scientific conduct include not only the pursuit of truth and the protection of the public interest, but also the various aspects of interpersonal conduct between scientists.

Researchers have a responsibility to the public, to funding agencies, and to professional colleagues to confront instances of possible misconduct when they arise. Such obligations are detailed in ethics guidelines for epidemiologists and other public health researchers.

The third case in this chapter is about a court case involving plagiarism of an epidemiologic study questionnaire. Researchers who invest time and effort in the development of a questionnaire do have a right to receive credit for their work and to control use of their instrument. On the other hand, the whole research enterprise stands to benefit if researchers share questionnaires and other research tools. Many excellent questionnaires have been developed through adaptation of questions used in previous studies. Although researchers may not have an obligation to share questionnaires with colleagues, the sharing of such research tools is consistent with the virtuous conduct of research. To ensure that conflicts do not arise, it is best to obtain permission before using questionnaires (or portions of them) developed by others.

Chapter 9: Publication and Interpretation of Research Findings

The first three cases in this chapter deal with issues of authorship including conflict over the order of coauthorship and honorary authorship. In the first case, a newly appointed assistant professor feels cheated of first-authorship credit. First authorship is generally extended to the individual who conceptualizes a research question, oversees the conduct of the study and the analysis, and takes primary responsibility for writing the results. In this situation, there was a lack of communication between the junior faculty member and the department chair about the expected time for completion of the manuscript and about who would draft the manuscript as first author. By failing to communicate effectively and by making herself first author while the assistant professor was on vacation, the department chair acted poorly as a mentor. On the other hand, research teams often are under pressure to be productive and to publish reports in a timely fashion. Both parties should have communicated their intentions about the manuscript, including who would be first author, early on.

In the second case, the conflict is again over the order of authorship. The role of the assistant professor in designing the study and supervising the graduate student would have justified first authorship if the assistant professor had also written most of the manuscript. Although the issue was resolved without substantial conflict in this case, such conflicts may require mediation by a third party such as a respected senior member of the faculty who has no interest in the outcome of the dispute.

The third case deals with claims to honorary coauthorship by a department head. To justify coauthorship of a scientific report, an individual (even a department head) must have made a contribution to the conceptualization of the research question and actual conduct of the research, and also must have assisted in preparing and approving the final report. The dubious practice of honorary coauthorship is inconsistent with the ethical conduct of research.

The fourth case in this chapter, involving pressure to go beyond the limits of the data, illustrates some of the difficult issues that can arise in multidisciplinary studies. Researchers have an obligation to communicate their work in ways that are understandable to others and to use sound judgment in interpreting their scientific findings. Of course, public health research does not take place in a societal vacuum. Researchers should take steps to respond to the needs of public policy makers and other stakeholders, while maintaining scientific objectivity and impartiality.

The next case has to do with questionable data analysis by a principal investigator. As this case illustrates, issues of scientific misconduct (dealt with in Chapter 6) also may arise in the publishing and interpreting of research findings. Ethics guidelines for epidemiologists and other health researchers outline responsibilities to professional colleagues and to society such as confronting or reporting improper behavior. The guidelines do not provide a detailed account of the specific steps that public health researchers should take in dealing with allegations of misconduct, however. Public health professionals may have to carefully analyze such situations when they arise and determine the best course of action using their own judgment and experience. Many institutions and agencies have policies for dealing with allegations of scientific misconduct or other improprieties.

The sixth case deals with the omission of out-of-range values in an environmental health study. Out-of-range or "high leverage" data points are sometimes omitted from analyses in order to improve the goodness-of-fit of statistical models. It is best to detail such omissions when reporting results, however, and to carry out the analyses with and without the out-of-range values, so that others can reach their own interpretations and conclusions.

Chapter 10: Communication Responsibilities of Public Health Professionals

The first case in this chapter deals with expert testimony on causation and the role of epidemiologists in court. Increasingly, epidemiologists are being called upon to provide expert testimony in courts of law about epidemiologic concepts and methods, including the strengths and limitations of various epidemiologic study designs. They also often are asked to give their opinion about the causes of certain diseases, based on the weight of the scientific data. In this case, the epidemiologist was asked if exposure to asbestos in the workplace was responsible for the observed cancer deaths, an issue fraught with uncertainty. In general, public health professionals should avoid overinter-preting the results of epidemiologic studies when communicating findings to other parties such as courts of law. There is a need to express measures of association and other statistical concepts (e.g, "borderline significance") in terms that lay persons can understand. The role of the epidemiologist as an expert witness is to answer questions honestly by expressing an impartial and objective opinion about the evidence regarding causation. One also should carefully explain the strengths and weaknesses of epidemiologic studies and the potential pitfalls of drawing causal inferences from observational data.

In the second case, a delay in the release of results from a study of childhood cancer is of concern. The researchers in this situation have an obligation to communicate the results of their study to members of the local community in a timely fashion. They acted responsibly by encouraging the funding agency to agree to the release of the findings so that the widest possible audience would stand to benefit from the research. Ideally, written agreements such as contracts between researchers and funding agencies should deal with such contingencies.

Similar issues are dealt with in the next two cases, which have to do with studies of dry-cleaning workers and heavy-metal contamination of produce. In general, researchers have a duty to inform participants of research results in a timely fashion and to avoid withholding information about potential health risks. This is true even when there is uncertainty about the seriousness or magnitude of the risks.

The careful checking of results and the submission of draft reports for rigorous scientific peer review are consistent with sound research practices. Such steps should be accomplished in an expeditious fashion, however, and unnecessary delays in informing participants about research findings should be avoided.

The fifth case has to do with the disclosure of information about asbestos health risks to the public. Public health education campaigns should be carefully planned so that they maximize potential benefits to members of the target population and to society, while minimizing risks. The principle of autonomy suggests that members of the targeted population should receive balanced and uncensored health information in understandable form, so that they can reach their own decisions about proper courses of action. The existence of scientific uncertainty about risks or about how best to minimize them is insufficient reason to withhold important health information from the public.

The last case in Chapter 10 has to do with media accounts of "mad cow disease" and consumer panic in Britain. As this case illustrates, public health professionals must use caution and sound judgment in communicating and interpreting health information. Both the public's right to know and the need to avoid overinterpretation of health information must be weighed in the balance. For example, when asked to provide an opinion about emerging patterns of disease or possible health hazards, public health professionals should point out areas of uncertainty or scientific agreement, and they must avoid overinterpreting the evidence. Differences in the ways scientists and lay persons evaluate and interpret risks also should be taken into account. For example, involuntary risks and those associated with dreaded diseases often are of greater concern to the public. In providing information to the news media, public health professionals can minimize adverse consequences and other risks by carefully preparing public statements and by checking to make sure that reporters understand the information conveyed to them.

Chapter 11: Public Health Practice

The first case in Chapter 11 has to do with ethical problems related to community concerns over contaminated ground water. The ethical considerations involved in decisions over whether to release test data for individual wells relate not only to rights to privacy and confidentiality, but also to the need to balance risks and potential benefits. Residents with contaminated wells could be harmed by the release of this information through a loss of property values. On the other hand, there is a need for residents to have adequate information so that they can assess the likelihood that their own wells will become contaminated. In situations like this, legal constraints and institutional policies often govern what information can or should be released by government agencies to outside parties. Public health scientists working on behalf of the community residents have an obligation to ensure that the data are adequately analyzed, perhaps through an independent analysis of the environmental risks.

Access to cancer chemotherapy protocols by the elderly is dealt with in the second case in this chapter. The equitable distribution of health care services such as chemotherapy protocols is grounded in the ethical principle of justice. Utilitarian theories of justice emphasize a mixture of criteria so that public utility is maximized. Because utilitarian approaches focus primarily on maximizing aggregate benefits, they can fail to consider adequately the final distribution of benefits to small subgroups of the population. Libertarian theories of justice, which hold that distributions of goods and services are best left to the marketplace, also provide little protection for underserved segments of the population. An egalitarian theory of justice implies that each person in society should share equally in the distribution of potential benefits.

As this case illustrates, when public health program planners are implementing interventions, they must consider the perspectives of community physicians and nurses so as to obtain sustained cooperation and support. When conflicts arise, they often can be resolved through a process of professional education and negotiation.

The third case involves risks and benefits of water chlorination in a particular community. Such public health questions often require careful health risk assessments. There also may be a need for additional epidemiologic studies to more adequately determine health risks and benefits in human populations. As this case illustrates, ethical considerations often underlie public policy formulation. In formulating such policies, public health professionals must determine how best to maximize benefits while minimizing risks.

Similar issues arise in the final case of this chapter, which has to do with a government program to control mosquito vectors for malaria. To evaluate the balance of risks and benefits, more information is needed about the adverse health effects of the pesticide exposure on women and children. One possible course of action would be to discontinue the pesticide program until the possible adverse health effects of the pesticide exposure are more adequately investigated. The question of who takes the risks while the natural experiment unfolds—so that scientists can be more certain—should be considered.

Chapter 12: Studies of Vulnerable Populations

The first case in this chapter is the Tuskegee Syphilis Study. This paradigmatic case in public health ethics illustrates the value of contemporary regulatory safeguards such as requirements for committee review and informed consent of participants. The medical and scientific communities often have failed to demonstrate that they are able to be effectively self-regulating in terms of ethical conduct. The responsibilities of researchers to participants in public health research studies (e.g., welfare protection, informed consent, privacy and confidentiality protection, and committee review) are outlined in proposed ethics guidelines for epidemiologists and other public health professionals. Vulnerable groups such as minority populations and individuals who are socioeconomically disadvantaged may be more susceptible to manipulative or coercive incentives.

The second case has to do with psychological risks posed by interviewing procedures in a case-control study of sudden infant death syndrome. It might be argued that any psychological distress resulting from participation in studies of this nature is likely to be relatively minor and transitory, and that the potential social benefits of the study also must be taken into account. Nevertheless, recently bereaved individuals and other vulnerable populations are deserving of protective measures to ensure that epidemiologic data are obtained in a less intrusive fashion.

The next case involves cancer control interventions aimed at children. The potential risks to the participants include local pain and infection from venipuncture. Other risks are social and legal and relate to potential breaches of confidentiality. Such risks can be minimized if the confidentiality of the information obtained in the study is rigorously protected. On balance, these risks are relatively minor and are outweighed by the potential benefits of the study. Since the effectiveness of the educational intervention has yet to be demonstrated, the use of a nonintervention control group appears to be acceptable. Ideally, the children randomly allocated to the control group would receive the educational intervention at the end of the study if the intervention is found to be effective. Children usually are considered minors until the age of 18 and need parental consent for most research-oriented activities. Researchers should further respect the autonomy of the minors by obtaining their assent to participation.

Additional ethical issues are raised in the last case in this chapter, a study of air pollution and asthma in African-American children. Although research protocols are commonly modified during the research process and many proposed studies are not funded, community partners may be unaware of these realities. Researchers should apprise their community partners of such possibilities and should avoid making promises they may not be able to keep. The investigators in this case had an obligation to notify the community clinics that the originally planned beneficial intervention was to be abandoned. By trying to obtain additional funds that would have made a community-based intervention possible, one investigator went further in trying to maximize the potential benefits of the study to the low-income clinics.

Chapter 13: Cross-Cultural Research

The first case in this chapter has to do with a study of sexually transmitted diseases in a periurban slum. The provision of free gynecological examinations and STD testing at the time of the first prenatal check-up is potentially manipulative in that women who might not otherwise agree to take part in the study might be manipulated into agreeing to do so. This is so because of the community's profound poverty. The release of the names of the women's sexual partners to local health workers might be required by local public health laws and statutes. The randomized study of male partners of the women treated for STDs raises justice-related concerns because of the lack of financial resources among residents of the community and the likelihood that many are unable to pay for costly prescription medications.

The second case, which has to do with an HIV vaccine trial in Africa, illustrates the difficult ethical problems that can arise when researchers from Western countries conduct trials of experimental vaccines or therapies in developing countries. Protocols for such vaccine trials should undergo committee review both in the investigator's home country and in the host country where the research is to be undertaken. Individuals and communities that bear the burden of experimental vaccine trials should stand to benefit from the research in case the vaccines are found to be safe and effective. In fact, many Africans will be unlikely to have access to costly vaccines for HIV.

The transcultural applicability of ethical standards such as provisions for obtaining the informed consent of participants remains controversial. Relativists argue that culturally sensitive standards are needed when studies are undertaken in other societies. Others argue convincingly that there is a need for a minimal set of universally applicable safeguards to protect the welfare and rights of individuals who are the target of health research.

The last case in this chapter has to do with a cancer control study of Native American women. To a greater or lesser extent, Native American women constitute a vulnerable population, particularly those who are pregnant, elderly, chronically ill, or poor. As such, they are deserving of added protections and safeguards against risks and potential harms posed by human subjects research.

There are no physical risks to the participants from taking part in the planned interview study. Some emotional distress may be experienced as a result of fear of cancer, embarrassment, or concerns over invasions of privacy. The social and legal risks posed by this study are primarily those that could result from the disclosure of confidential information. Such risks should be minimized by strict adherence to confidentiality safeguards for all information collected.

Both the nature of the research and the choice of interview sites influence the likelihood of such risks. For example, it may be more difficult to maintain privacy in home interviews as compared with telephone interviews. Participation in focus-group sessions on sensitive topics such as sexual history also may call unwanted attention to women. In the planned study, such concerns should be addressed by limiting topics for discussion in the focus-group sessions to less-sensitive topics, and through the use of telephone interviews for the structured interviews to the extent feasible.

Special confidentiality concerns are raised by the use of the exhaustive list of heads of households maintained by the Tribal

Council for use in sampling potential respondents. Such tribal rolls play an important role in tribal cohesiveness and communication. The inadvertent release of this mailing list to a third party could have serious consequences for the Indian Nation. Researchers privileged to make use of such tribal rolls have a special obligation to maintain their security and confidentiality.

Potential benefits to the participants and to the Indian Nation are more likely to be maximized by participatory research that is collaborative and empowering. The investigators addressed such concerns by involving members of the Tribal Council in the planning of the study and through the planned use of Native American interviewers.

Participants in the planned study and future generations of Native American women may ultimately benefit from a possible reduction in breast and cervical cancer risk. The Native American community also may be left with an increased capacity for carrying out health needs assessments as well as useful information that may help overcome barriers to cancer screening services.

The informed consent of each participant should be obtained verbally before interview data are obtained. An additional safeguard is the provision for obtaining the consent and cooperation of community leaders, who are members of the Tribal Council, before undertaking the study. The Tribal Council members should serve as a community advisory board throughout the conduct of the research.

The Native American women who are being included in the study are being specifically targeted because they represent an underserved and possibly high-risk population that has been understudied.

Chapter 14: Genetic Research and Testing

The first case in this chapter involves screening for genetic markers of cancer risk. Members of cancer-prone families should undergo genetic testing only if the potential benefits outweigh the risks. In this case, risks include discrimination by insurance companies or future employers and possible adverse psychological effects. Public health professionals can minimize such risks by rigorously protecting the confidentiality of the genetic information and by advocating for improved regulatory protections. The provision of psychological counseling services also may be important. On the other hand, genetic testing for the $p53$ mutation may facilitate early detection of cancer. Nevertheless, children are less likely to be in a position to make an autonomous, informed choice about whether or not to undergo the testing. For this reason, some ethicists have argued that such testing of children for genetic markers of cancer risk should ideally be delayed until they are older and can better reach their own decisions.

The next case has to do with genetic testing for BRCA1 or BRCA2 mutations in women in the general population. The risks of such genetic testing include the possibility of discrimination based solely on a women's genotype and the inadvertent release of test results to a third party. Strict confidentiality safeguards are needed to minimize risks and harms from the release of genetic information to a third party. The adequacy of informed consent also should be addressed.

Ethical issues also are raised by the notification of women who undergo genetic testing about their own risks of cancer. Knowledge of genetic predisposition to a disease may lead to feelings of inadequacy, fear, or depression, which may result in impaired psychological health. There should be some provision for providing appropriate counseling for women who test positive for BRCA1 or BRCA2 mutations.

Ethical considerations underlie the choice of a research hypothesis and decisions about what research studies to undertake. Of concern are how best to allocate scarce resources (in this case, resources for cancer control research) and how to maximize potential benefits of the research while minimizing risks. Cancer control researchers have responsibilities to protect the public's health and to advance the field while respecting the rights and welfare of the populations they study.

The last case in this chapter illustrates some of the pitfalls of genetic screening in the workplace. Instead of encouraging companies to implement engineering controls to reduce workplace exposures, the emphasis is placed on identifying workers who are relatively susceptible to environmental exposures. Workers who are found to be more susceptible to such exposures may unfairly lose their jobs or be moved to less lucrative positions away from potentially hazardous areas. Companies stand to benefit from such genetic screening by reducing future compensation claims for work-related illnesses.

Other issues relate to the question of who should control access to such genetic test results. Ideally, control should rest with the workers or their private physicians rather than with company officials. Workers have a right to receive information about their own test results, even if the prognostic accuracy of the genetic tests is unknown or uncertain.

Chapter 15: HIV/AIDS Prevention and Treatment

The first case in this chapter is about ethical and public policy issues surrounding HIV antibody home testing. Such home test kits may increase access to HIV antibody testing while protecting privacy and freedom of choice. By potentially increasing the number of persons who know their own HIV antibody seropositivity status, the introduction of HIV home testing may contribute to efforts to combat the AIDS epidemic by slowing the transmission of HIV in the population. On the other hand, individuals who learn at home that they are HIV antibody positive, in the absence of immediate counseling services, may be at increased risk for suicide, anxiety, or depression. The purpose of federal regulations and statutes on prescription drugs and medical devices, such as policies governing the use of home test kits, is to protect the public from ineffective or harmful products. Libertarians view restrictive policies of FDA or other government agencies as overly paternalistic or intrusive.

The second case has to do with the high cost of combination therapy with antiretroviral drugs and issues of distributive justice. The equitable distribution of health care products such as antiretroviral drugs, both between countries and within individual nations, is grounded in the ethical principle of justice. Libertarian theories of justice, which hold that distributions of goods and services are best left to the marketplace, provide little protection for socioeconomically disadvantaged populations in countries around the world. Under an egalitarian theory of justice, which implies that each person in society should share equally in the distribution of potential benefits, those who are least well-off also stand to benefit from public services and products such as new AIDS therapies. Such issues related to the allocation of scarce resources are dealt with further in Chapter 16.

The third case in this chapter has to do with a trial of AZT in the prevention of vertical transmission of HIV from mother to child. A number of ethical issues were addressed by the investigators in designing the study. For example, the investigators had to consider whether the potential benefits to the women and their infants outweighed the risks. They also had to consider whether the choice of a target population (mostly Latin and African-American women) was equitable in terms of the distribution of risks and potential benefits. In this situation, minority women were specifically targeted because of their increased risk of HIV infection and AIDS and not because they were a convenient choice for the investigators. The monetary and other incentives provided to these low-income women may be deemed reasonable in relation to the burdens of taking part in the study, and not overly manipulative or coercive.

Chapter 16: Allocation of Scarce Resources and Health Care Reform

The first case in Chapter 16 is about health maintenance organization (HMO) contracts. So-called "gag rules" in some HMO contracts, which were outlawed by the federal government in the United States in 1996, represent conflicting interests; such rules contravened the responsibilities of physicians to fully inform their patients about treatment options, to disclose financial incentives that encourage the physicians to limit care, and to always act in the best interests of each individual patient. Generally, disclosures about which treatments are covered and other benefits and financial arrangements are made in brochures or booklets distributed by HMOs to potential enrollees and individuals covered by the plan. Physicians do have an obligation to provide key information about treatment options at the time service is rendered.

The next case is about health care for undocumented aliens. Public policies that require health care providers to report suspected illegal aliens may contribute to the spread of communicable diseases such as tuberculosis by deterring illegal aliens from seeking health care. Such communicable diseases often are detected through case finding when individuals are treated for unrelated illnesses at public clinics.

The last case, which concerns cancer screening in socioeconomically disadvantaged populations, also raises issues of distributive justice. The principle of justice informs decisions about how much of the community-based organization's resources should be devoted to cancer prevention in socioeconomically disadvantaged populations. Utilitarian theories of justice can fail to ensure distribution of benefits to small population subgroups. Libertarian theories of justice, which hold that distributions of goods and services are best left to the marketplace, also provide little protection for underserved segments of the population. An egalitarian theory of justice implies that each person in society should share equally in the distribution of potential benefits.

In determining whether an educational program or mass media campaign is acceptable to the target population, a form of community consent from representatives of the underserved population, such as community leaders, would be desirable. A community advisory committee, consisting of individuals from the targeted population, should provide input and feedback throughout the planning and conduct of the program.

Suggestions for Further Reading

Arnold, R. M., Povar, G. J. & Howell, J. D. (1987). The humanities, humanistic behavior, and the humane physician: A cautionary note. *Ann Int Med,* 106, 313-318.

Bebeau, M. J. & Brabeck, M. M. (1987). Integrating care and justice issues in professional moral education: A general perspective. *J Moral Education,* 16, 189-203.

Burling, S. J., Lumley, J. S., McCarthy, L. S., et al. (1990). Review of the teaching of medical ethics in London medical schools. *J Med Ethics,* 16, 206-209.

Coughlin, S. S. (1996). Advancing professional ethics in epidemiology. *J Epidemiol Biostat,* 1, 71-77.

Coughlin, S. S. & Etheredge, G. D. (1995). On the need for ethics curricula in epidemiology. *Epidemiology, 6*, 566-567.

Coughlin, S. S. & Etheredge, G. D. (1995). Teaching ethics and epidemiology: Initial experiences at two schools of public health. *Epidemiology Monitor, 16*, 5-7.

Coughlin, S. S., Etheredge, G. D., Metayer, C. & Martin, S. A., Jr. (1996). Remember Tuskegee: Public health student knowledge of the ethical significance of the Tuskegee Syphilis Study. *Am J Prev Med, 12*, 242-246.

Fox, E., Arnold, R. M. & Brody, B. (1995). Medical ethics education: Past, present, and future. *Acad Med, 70*, 761-769.

Friedman, P. J. (1990). Research ethics: A teaching agenda for academic medicine [Commentary]. *Acad Med, 65*, 32-33.

Friedman, P. J. (Ed.). (1993). Integrity in biomedical research [Special issue]. *Acad Med, 68*(Suppl.).

Gilmer, P. J. (1995). Teaching science at the university level: What about the ethics? *Science and Engineering Ethics, 1*, 173-180.

Goodman, K. W. & Prineas, R. J. (1996). Toward an ethics curriculum in epidemiology. In S. S. Coughlin & T. L. Beauchamp (Eds.). *Ethics and epidemiology*. (pp. 290-303). New York: Oxford University Press.

Gunsalus, C. K. (1993). Institutional structures to ensure research integrity. *Acad Med, 68*(Suppl.), S33-S38.

Hafferty, F. W. & Franks, R. (1994). The hidden curriculum, ethics teaching, and the structure of medical education. *Acad Med, 69*, 861-871.

Korenman, S. G. & Shipp, A. C. (1994). *Teaching the responsible conduct of research through a case study approach. A handbook for instructors.* Washington, DC: Association of American Medical Colleges.

LaPidus, J. B. & Mishkin, B. (1990). Values and ethics in the graduate education of scientists. In W. W. May (Ed.), *Ethics and higher education* (pp. 238-298). New York: Macmillan Publishing Co.

Macrina, F. L. (1995). *Scientific integrity. An introductory text with cases.* Washington, DC: American Society for Microbiology Press.

Mitchell, K. R., Lovat, T. J. & Myser, C. M. (1992). Teaching bioethics to medical students: The Newcastle experience. *Med Educ, 26*, 290-300.

Mitchell, K. R., Myser, C. & Kerridge, I. H. (1993). Assessing the clinical ethical competence of undergraduate medical students. *J Med Ethics*, 19, 230-236.

Pellegrino, E. D. (1989). Teaching medical ethics: Some persistent questions and some responses. *Acad Med*, 64, 701-703.

Pellegrino, E. D., Hart, R. J., Henderson, S. R., et al. (1985). Relevance and utility of courses in medical ethics. A survey of physicians' perceptions. *JAMA*, 253, 49-53.

Penslar, R. L. (Ed.). (1996). *Research ethics. Cases & materials.* Indianapolis, IA: Indiana University Press.

Rossignol, A. M. & Goodmonson, S. (1996). Are ethical topics in epidemiology included in the graduate epidemiology curricula? *Am J Epidemiol*, 142, 1265-1268.

Sachs, G. A. & Siegler, M. (1993). Teaching scientific integrity and the responsible conduct of research. *Acad Med*, 68, 871-875.

Self, D. J., Wolinsky, F. D. & Baldwin, D. C. (1989). The effect of teaching medical ethics on medical students' moral reasoning. *Acad Med*, 64, 755-759.

Sulmasy, D. P., Geller, G., Levine, D. M., et al. (1990). Medical house officers' knowledge, attitudes, and confidence regarding medical ethics. *Arch Intern Med*, 150, 2509-2513

Sulmasy, D. P., Geller, G., Levine, D. M. & Faden, R. R. (1993). A randomized trial of ethics education for medical house officers. *J Med Ethics*, 19, 157-163.

Index